BIOSENSORS

Biosensors

Theory and Applications

DONALD G. BUERK, Ph.D.

INSTITUTE FOR ENVIRONMENTAL MEDICINE
UNIVERSITY OF PENNSYLVANIA
PHILADELPHIA, PENNSYLVANIA

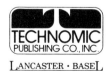

TECHNOMIC
PUBLISHING CO., INC.
LANCASTER · BASEL

Biosensors
a **TECHNOMIC**®publication

Published in the Western Hemisphere by
Technomic Publishing Company, Inc.
851 New Holland Avenue
Box 3535
Lancaster, Pennsylvania 17604 U.S.A.

Distributed in the Rest of the World by
Technomic Publishing AG

Printed in the United States of America
10 9 8 7 6 5 4 3 2 1

Main entry under title:
  Biosensors: Theory and Applications

A Technomic Publishing Company book
Bibliography: p.
Includes index p. 213

Library of Congress Card No. 92-61490
ISBN No. 0-87762-975-7

To my loving wife, Steffie,
whose moral support and spiritual understanding kept me going,
and to my sons, Jesse and Daniel,
whose love and encouragement made the effort worthwhile.

TABLE OF CONTENTS

CHAPTER 1

Introduction

A biosensor may be broadly defined as any measuring device that contains a biological element. A schematic drawing for a generalized biosensor is shown in Figure 1.1. A target analyte (illustrated by solid circles) in the external medium must be able to enter the biosensor. The external membrane of the biosensor must be permeable to the analyte, and if possible, exclude other chemical species that the biosensor might also be sensitive to. The biological element inside the biosensor then interacts with the analyte and responds in some manner that can be detected by a transducer. The biological element may convert the analyte to another chemical species (represented by open circles) through a biochemical reaction; produce or release another chemical product in response to the analyte stimulus; change its optical, electrical or mechanical properties; or make some other response that can be reliably quantified. There may be another internal membrane near the transducer which might have different permeability properties than the external membrane. The output signal from a biosensor depends on the type of transducer it uses. The transducer may be a conventional electrochemical sensor, or may be based on another technology.

This book is an overview of the basic theories of operation for a number of specific types of biosensor transducers that have been investigated, with a general survey of some of the many applications using various biological elements that have been tested to date. A major portion of this book has been devoted to electrochemical transducers, since they have been most widely used. In Chapter 2, the theories for operating electrochemical transducers, including amperometric (current), potentiometric (voltage), and coulometric (charge) techniques will be described. Basic theories for conventional electrodes that measure pH, O_2, and other chemical analytes will be discussed further in Chapter 3. Modifications of these conventional

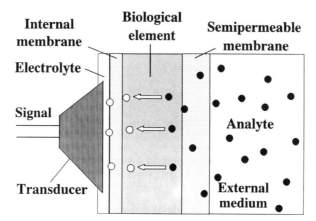

FIGURE 1.1. *General principles for a biosensor. The specific chemical target (analyte) is recognized by the biological element, creating a stimulus to the detecting transducer from which a reproducible signal is measured.*

electrodes by enzymes will be described in Chapter 4. Miniaturization techniques for electrochemical devices are discussed in Chapter 5. Optical technology will be discussed in Chapter 6, and other technologies in Chapter 7. The rapidly developing field of immunosensors, which allows detection of analytes by very highly specific molecular recognition, is surveyed in Chapter 8. Biosensors using a wide panorama of living biological elements are surveyed in Chapter 9. Finally, Chapter 10 discusses some areas where there are likely to be important applications for commercial biosensors in the near future.

1.1 BRIEF HISTORICAL BACKGROUND

One of the many landmark achievements in our modern era of scientific discovery was the understanding of acid/base chemistry. The Danish scientist Sørenson (1909) described his experimental procedures for determining hydrogen ion (H^+) concentration, defined the concept of pH, and standardized the pH scale. Furthermore, he investigated the effect of pH on rates of enzymatic hydrolysis. He correctly concluded that pH had very important effects on chemical and biochemical processes. By the early 1900s, the concept of electrochemical potential differences due to oxidation and reduction reactions was beginning to be recognized and the theory further refined. The hydrogen gas (H_2) electrode system, consisting of a platinum (Pt) electrode with an electrodeposit of Pt black to increase its surface area, became the standard for electrochemical measurements. The reduction/oxidation (redox) potential for H^+/H_2 was defined as zero.

The new technology was quickly adopted for biological measurements. Michaelis and Davidoff (1912) used a Pt/H_2 pH electrode to measure the pH of lysed red blood cells. Using the same system, Michaelis and Kramsztyk (1914) measured pH in various mammalian tissues immediately after dissection, then later after boiling the tissues. Buytendijk (1927) was the first to use a solid metal antimony pH electrode for medical purposes. Today, the measurement of blood pH is a vital and routine clinical measurement, and we understand how important a role the H^+ ion plays in respiration and metabolism. Even so, there are still many unanswered questions with regard to the regulation of acid-base balance in the whole organism, in individual organs, and at the single-cell level. Also, there are many new types of pH sensors still under development using a variety of different technologies.

Another landmark achievement in science this century was the development of modern electrochemistry. Important new electrochemical techniques were discovered by Heyrovsky (1922) in the early part of this century in Prague, Czechoslovakia. He developed an instrument that used the surface of a growing drop of mercury to measure oxidation and reduction potentials for a number of different chemical species. This chemical sensor became known as a dropping mercury electrode polarograph. The electrode surface was formed by a continuous, slow stream of mercury through a glass tube, which formed a spherical drop that eventually dropped from the end. The mercury was recycled. A number of practical applications for the dropping mercury electrode polarograph were developed in his laboratory. During a visit to Stanford University in 1933, Heyrovsky presented his polarograph results to scientists in the United States. Subsequently, a large number of investigators began using this new electrochemical technology. Heyrovsky was the recipient of the Nobel Prize for chemistry in 1959 in recognition of his pioneering work.

Some of the early research using this technology was directed to measurements of O_2 concentrations in several different biological media. By monitoring the current from the dropping mercury electrode with a sensitive galvanometer, Müller and Baumberger (1935) measured O_2 in biological fluids. Their instrumentation allowed them to make more accurate measurements than previous scientists had been able to make. They found that the partial pressure (PO_2) in fluids could be measured within $\pm 1\%$ accuracy in the range from 10^{-3} to 1 atmosphere (1 atm = 760 mmHg = 101.3 kPa). Later, Baumberger (1938) used the dropping mercury electrode polarograph to determine the oxyhemoglobin equilibrium curve for O_2. Also, he was the first to measure skin PO_2. In another biological application, Petering and Daniels (1938) used the mercury polarograph to measure O_2 consumption rates for algae, yeast, and blood cells. Beecher et al. (1942) attempted to use the polarograph clinically.

One of the major advantages of the dropping mercury electrode was that the surface was continually being renewed with each drop. Thus the detecting element was always fresh and did not depend on the prior history of measurements. However, there were a number of technical difficulties encountered by scientists using the dropping mercury electrode and large measurement artifacts were possible. The polarograph was not always stable for sufficiently long time periods, and required frequent calibrations. Electrode fouling was the most severe problem, and the mercury often needed to be cleaned before it could be reused for another measurement. Also, relatively large samples were required for the analysis, and the sample needed to be well mixed. Vibrating or rotating electrode systems were designed to maximize convective transport to the sensor. A significant drawback of the dropping mercury electrode for biological studies was the inherent toxicity of mercury to living organisms. It soon became clear that better measurement techniques were needed.

1.2 EARLY APPLICATIONS FOR NOBLE METAL ELECTRODES

The first steps towards the development of O_2 sensors began nearly a century ago in Göttingen, Germany. Ludwig Danneel (1897, 1898) scientifically investigated the current generated between two large Pt electrodes held at a 20 mV potential difference. The resulting current was found to be linear with O_2 concentration, but instabilities were observed and difficulties in making biological measurements were reported. Glasstone (1931) investigated the use of Pt electrodes for polarographic measurements in Heyrovsky's laboratory. Although he obtained favorable results, this technique did not receive as much early attention due to the success of Heyrovsky's polarograph.

Blinks and Skow (1938) replaced the dropping mercury electrode with Pt electrodes, and were successful in measuring O_2 evolution by algae during photosynthesis. They found a current-voltage plateau for O_2 in the polarization voltage range from -0.3 to -0.7 V (Pt cathode negative relative to the anode). They were the first to demonstrate that the limiting current at a constant voltage within this plateau range was linear with O_2 concentration from 0 to 99.5 % O_2. Their bare cathode electrode had a response time of < 1 second. Further development of the polarographic method using gold (Au) and Pt metal electrodes took place during World War II in the laboratories of the Johnson Foundation at the University of Pennsylvania in Philadelphia. The principal scientists involved in this work were Philip Davies, Detlov Bronk, and Frank Brink, Jr. They were particularly interested in using O_2 electrodes to investigate O_2 metabolism of the brain and nervous system. To achieve the spatial resolution needed for meaningful physiological measurements, Davies and Brink (1942) developed the first true O_2 microelectrodes. However, the bare noble metal O_2 electrodes usually suffered from a gradual loss of sensitivity when exposed to blood and tissue, and measurement artifacts were encountered.

It was not until the modifications by Clark (1956), that the electrochemical detection of O_2 was reliably made. The Clark O_2 electrode has subsequently led to a period of rapid growth for biosensor applications in the medical and biological fields. A schematic drawing of the Clark electrode design will be shown in Chapter 3, along with a discussion of the general theory of O_2 electrodes. The simple modification that made this sensor more reliable than bare cathodes was the physical isolation of the cathode from the measurement medium. This was accomplished by placing a gas-permeable membrane over the cathode. The cathode was either a Pt or Au wire sealed in glass, with an Ag/AgCl wire anode. An electrolyte solution, typically 2 M KCl, was placed inside the body of the electrode housing to complete the electrical circuit between the anode and cathode. Early tests in blood, plasma, urine, and other solutions were successfully made using a polypropylene membrane. The Clark O_2 electrode quickly led to other research efforts that marked the birth of biosensor technology. As will be discussed further in Chapters 4 and 5, the Clark O_2 electrode and similar membrane-covered electrodes are vital components of many biosensors in current use.

1.3 EARLY OPTICAL METHODS

Britton Chance (1991) has recently reviewed the development of modern optical methods, especially with regard to spectrophotometric measurements in tissue. He also presented a historical perspective on the evolution of optical techniques beginning with the early work by Otto Warburg in Germany before World War II. Advances in electronics that had been made during World War II were successfully applied to optical instrumentation by Britton Chance at the University of Pennsylvania, Franz Jöbsis-VanderVliet at Duke University, Dietrich Lübbers in Germany, and many other scientists. The principle of using a differential, dual beam spectrophotometer had been developed by the English physicist John Tyndall in the late 1800s. This concept was applied to biological measurements by several laboratories, and a modified split beam spectrophotometer made commercially by

Beckman Instruments became an important optical instrument in many laboratories. Multiple channel devices for simultaneous scanning of more than one wavelength were designed and improved upon. A wide range of optical methods have become well accepted for biophysical and biochemical measurements. These techniques have also been adopted for use as optical transducers in biosensors.

1.4 IDEAL BIOSENSOR CHARACTERISTICS

The optimum design of electrochemical, optical, and other types of biosensors is dictated by several basic physical properties of the measuring system, as well as those of the media in which the measurement is made. Some of the most pertinent properties and characteristic behaviors of ideal biosensors are listed as follows.

1.4.1 Sensitivity

The sensitivity is usually defined as the final steady state change in the magnitude of the biosensor output signal with respect to the change in concentration of a specific chemical species ($\Delta S / \Delta C$), as illustrated in Figure 1.2. The target analyte is usually not directly detected by the biosensor. More often, changes in concentration of a co-reactant or co-product of a chemical reaction taking place within the biosensor are measured. The sensitivity of the biosensor with respect to the chemical substrate of interest

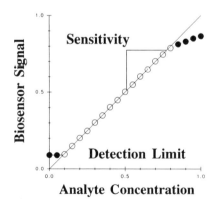

FIGURE 1.2. *Calibration curve for a biosensor with a linear range (open circles), showing lower limit of detection and nonlinear behavior at higher concentration (solid circles). Sensitivity is defined as the slope of the linear range ($\Delta S / \Delta C$).*

(the analyte) must then be related to the directly detected chemical species through the appropriate stoichiometry of the chemical reaction. In other cases, some physical property has been altered by the biological element, which is then measured by the transducer.

For some biosensor types, measurements are based on the dynamic response of the biosensor. Sensitivity may be defined in this situation as the change in the signal with time for a given change in concentration ($\Delta S / \Delta t / \Delta C$), or some other relationship that depends on time. Time integration, frequency analysis, or other data processing of the time varying signals may also be of value in relating them to the concentration of the analyte.

There are many factors that determine the effective sensitivity of a given biosensor design to a target analyte. These include the physical size of the sensor, the thickness of the membranes and resulting mass transport of chemical species from the sample to the sensing region, and various processes that deactivate the biosensor or otherwise impair its operation over time. Ideally, the sensitivity of a given biosensor should remain constant during its lifetime and should be sufficiently high to allow convenient measurement of the transducer output signal with electronic instrumentation.

1.4.2 Calibration

An ideal biosensor should be easily calibrated simply by exposing it to prepared standard solutions or gases containing different known concentrations of the target analyte. Calibration curves need not require many data points to obtain the sensitivity, especially if the operational behavior of the biosensor is known. Calibration points should bracket the range of values that will be measured, to avoid possibly unreliable extrapolations outside the expected range. Ideally, it should be necessary to perform a calibration procedure only one time to determine the sensitivity of the biosensor for subsequent measurements. In practical terms, however, it is usually necessary to make periodic calibrations at regular intervals to characterize changes in the sensitivity with time.

1.4.3 Linearity

A perfectly linear biosensor will have a constant sensitivity over the concentration range from zero to the maximum substrate concentration that can be physically dissolved in the measurement medium. Practically, the region of linearity may be restricted to a narrower range of substrate concentrations, as represented by the open circles in Figure 1.2. A two point calibration can be made anywhere in the linear range, allowing the measurements in this range to be reliably converted to accurate substrate concentrations.

A biosensor need not be linear to be practically useful, as long as the calibration curve can be obtained with sufficient accuracy to interpret the biosensor signal. One correction is to approximate any nonlinearities as a series of linear regions. Some biosensors have semi-logarithmic sensitivities ($\Delta S / \Delta \ln C$) which are predicted from the chemical principles on which they operate. Although these sensors may be classified as nonlinear, the signals can be readily linearized by replotting on a semi-logarithmic scale. The logarithmic relationship would be obtained with all similar biosensors, with minor differences in sensitivities. Other nonlinear relationships can be used as long as an adequate number of points on the calibration curve are obtained to accurately characterize the variable sensitivity of the biosensor. If each biosensor has a unique, nonlinear calibration curve, it still may be practically useful, but will require more complicated signal analysis to extract the desired information.

1.4.4 Limit of Detection

Ideally, the lowest concentration of substrate that can be detected by a biosensor (shown in Figure 1.2) should be limited only by the resolution of the electronic instrumentation used for the measurement. In practical terms, other considerations cause the lower limit of detection to be higher. For example, electrochemical transducers using potentiometric measurements may have interference from other ions and surface reactions that limit the measurement. Obviously, the range of expected analyte concentra-

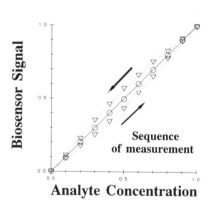

FIGURE 1.3. *Calibration curves for an ideal biosensor (open circles) and one with hysteresis (open triangles). In the latter case, the previous history of the measurement affects subsequent readings. The sequence and timing of the measurements (arrows) determines how much deviation from ideal behavior is encountered.*

tions for an intended application must be detectable in order for the biosensor to be useful.

1.4.5 Background Signal

Usually, a biosensor signal will have some background level that must be subtracted. The background signal may make the determination of the lower limit of detection for a biosensor difficult to determine accurately. Current leakage, small potential differences in the electronic instrumentation or due to dissimilar metal to metal contacts in the wire leads of the biosensor, or electrochemical factors could be responsible for the background signal. The background signal is not electrical noise. For a linear system, the true signal is simply

$$S = S_{measured} - S_{background} \tag{1}$$

For a semi-logarithmic signal, it is more convenient to refer to a measurement at a reference concentration C_{ref}

$$\frac{S}{S_{ref}} = \ln \frac{\text{biosensor measurement} - \text{background}}{\text{reference measurement} - \text{background}} \tag{2}$$

where either the natural ($\ln$) or base 10 logarithm ($\log_{10}$) can be used. The above relationships assume that the background signal remains constant as the biosensor signal changes, but this may not always be true.

1.4.6 Hysteresis

An ideal biosensor should not be affected by its past history of measurements, and would have zero hysteresis, as represented by the straight line through the open circles in Figure 1.3. However, energy can be absorbed, or the local chemical environment can be changed during a measurement, which would then have an effect on the next measurement. This is illustrated by the deviation from the ideal shown by the open triangles in Figure 1.3, for a sequence of measurements taken in the order indicated by the two arrows. For example, a measurement made at a high analyte concentration might be accompanied by a pH change in the sensor electrolyte solution. If the pH has not been adequately buffered in this solution, the next measurement made at a low analyte concentration could be affected. This could be a problem with an enzyme-based biosensor where the enzyme activity is strongly pH dependent. Another possibility is that during the measurement period at high concentrations, the analyte could diffuse into the biosensor.

If a second measurement at low concentration is made, the accumulated analyte in the biosensor could then diffuse back out until equilibrium is reached with the external sample. If the sample volume is small, this could have a large effect on the final steady state measurement. Hysteresis could also affect the transient responses of the biosensor. In some cases, hysteresis can be minimized by making slow changes.

1.4.7 Drift and Long-Term Stability

An ideal biosensor should have constant sensitivity for its entire lifetime, or at least during the time that measurements are being made. There are a multitude of factors that can reduce the sensitivity, such as oxide formation on the electrode, and "fouling" or "poisoning" by direct adsorption of proteins or other chemical substrates on the membrane or on the sensor surface. It is usually necessary to recalibrate the biosensor at frequent intervals during its use, so that the signal can be corrected for the drift in sensitivity with time.

A hypothetical example for a transducer with a 20% loss in sensitivity over a measurement period is illustrated in Figure 1.4. Three time courses for the possible change in sensitivity are shown [curves (a), (b), (c)] at the top of Figure 1.4, including a linear decrease (b). The uncorrected signal is shown at the bottom, along with the appropriate corrections for drift. It is always simplest to assume that the drift is approximately linear with time between calibrations, but errors can result, as shown. The greatest error

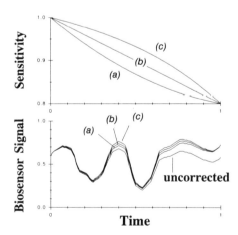

FIGURE 1.4. *Effect of 20% loss in sensitivity (top panel) with uncorrected drift in biosensor signal (bottom panel). Three different time courses for loss in sensitivity are illustrated [(a), (b), (c)], with corresponding corrections to biosensor signal.*

would be near the midpoint of the measurement if the drift is linear. However, it is also possible to have sudden, step-like changes in sensitivity. These might be caused by mechanical or chemical events. In this case, the time when the shift occurred may be difficult to identify and a linear correction factor would not be justified. If the event can be identified, it may be possible to assume constant, but different sensitivities before and after it occurs to correct the signal. It is also possible to have a transient change in sensitivity that would not be detected, for example by the temporary deposit of a film over the biosensor. The film could be washed away upon recalibration, with the biosensor returning back to its original sensitivity.

1.4.8 Selectivity (Interference)

The ideal biosensor will only respond to changes in concentration of the target analyte, and will not be influenced by the presence of other chemical species. Otherwise, false readings for the analyte concentration would be obtained if it is actually the concentration of the interfering species that is changing. If it is not possible to control the concentration of the interfering species, then it will be necessary to measure it with another type of chemical transducer in order to correct the composite signal from the biosensor. There are also other factors, for example pH, where the chemical reaction is altered. This might be considered to be an indirect form of interference. As will be discussed later for individual applications, there have been many approaches for designing biosensors to reduce interference and improve the selectivity for measuring the desired analyte.

1.4.9 Dynamic Response

The physical properties and relative size of a biosensor probe determine how quickly it will respond to a change in concentration of the target analyte it measures. The principal mechanism is usually simple diffusion of the chemical species from the sample to the active surface of the transducer. The mass flux of the target analyte and/or the reactant that is being detected is proportional to the concentration differences, the effective diffusion coefficients D_{eff} for each species moving through the different elements of the sensor (membranes, electrolytes, and other structures), and the thickness of each element. This type of response is often referred to as being dependent on a diffusion-limited process.

1.4.10 Planar Membrane

Analytical solutions can be derived from theoretical models for biosensors with different geometries and simple boundary conditions. For example, larger electrodes are often modeled as a planar element covered with a simple, uniform membrane of finite thickness (L). Simple diffusion theory

$$\frac{\partial C}{\partial t} = -D \frac{\partial^2 C}{\partial x^2} \tag{3}$$

can be applied to a chemical species (C) moving through the membrane with a diffusivity (D), or to the partial pressure (P) of a dissolved gas

$$\frac{\partial P}{\partial t} = -D \frac{\partial^2 P}{\partial x^2} \tag{4}$$

through Henry's law of solubility $(C = \alpha P)$, where α is the solubility coefficient.

The normalized time response for a signal, $f(t)$, changing from an initial value, f_0, to a final value, f_1, following the step change in concentration of substrate on the outer surface is given by an infinite series solution

$$\frac{f(t) - f_0}{f_1 - f_0} = 1 + 2 \sum_{n=1}^{\infty} (-1)^n \exp^{-(n^2 t / \tau_{\text{eff}})} \tag{5}$$

where an effective time scaling factor τ_{eff} can be defined as

$$\tau_{\text{eff}} = \frac{L^2}{\pi^2 D_{\text{eff}}} \tag{6}$$

The dynamic response for a planar membrane is shown in Figure 1.5 as a function of the dimensionless time (t/τ_{eff}) following a sudden (step change) increase or decrease in substrate on the outer membrane surface. A single term in the series can be used to accurately describe the final 50% of the response (solid curve at right of Figure 1.5), but many more terms are required for the initial part of the step. The first 2% of the response is shown in the left panel. The response calculated from the series solution with 20 terms is shown by a dotted line in both right and left panels. Below $t/\tau_{\text{eff}} = 1$, the single term drastically underestimates the step response. The series solution with three terms (dashed line, left panel) would give a very good representation of the step response for the range from 2% to 100%. The membrane causes an effective delay in the initial response for about $t/\tau_{\text{eff}} = 0.3$, where little change can be seen in this time period (left panel).

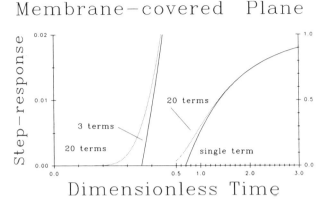

FIGURE 1.5. *Series solution for time response due to diffusion following a step change in concentration [Equation (5), planar membrane].*

1.4.11 Spherical Membrane

Similarly, an analytical solution can be found for diffusion through a uniform membrane in spherical coordinates. This modeling approach is often used for microelectrodes, where the tip of the sensor is very small compared to the external measuring medium. The dynamic response is

$$\frac{f(t) - f_0}{f_1 - f_0} = 1 - 4\sqrt{\frac{\tau_{\text{eff}}}{\pi t}} \sum_{n=0}^{\infty} \exp^{-(2n+1)^2(\tau_{\text{eff}}/t)} \tag{7}$$

with an effective time scaling factor

$$\tau_{\text{eff}} = \frac{(d_m - d_0)^2}{D_{\text{eff}}} \tag{8}$$

where the membrane diameter is d_m and electrode diameter d_0, for a total membrane thickness $L = d_m - d_0$. The step response is illustrated in Figure 1.6, and is nearly 83% complete in one dimensionless time unit. As can be seen, the analytical solution with only one term in the infinite series (solid curve, left panel) is quite good over the range from 0% to 95%. Using only two terms (middle panel) extends the range out to 99.5% with reasonably good accuracy. For the final 0.5%, more terms are required. The series solution with three terms is shown (dashed line, right panel).

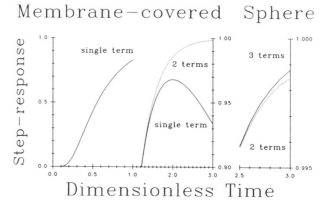

FIGURE 1.6. *Series solution for time response due to spherical diffusion [Equation (7), membrane-covered sphere].*

Analytical solutions have also been determined for cylindrical coordinates, using series solutions with Bessel functions to model the response. Further details of mass transport modeling for various boundary conditions and geometries can be found in the book by Crank (1956).

1.4.12 Flow Sensitivity

In some situations, convective transport of substrate to the outer membrane of the sensor may become important. Such processes are often referred to as being flow-limited. Significant hydrodynamic boundary layers may exist in the flowing medium near the biosensor. Mathematical analyses become more complicated, perhaps requiring numerical solutions in many cases. However, empirical engineering correlations (for example with Reynolds number) are possible. In these systems, generally the response time will decrease as flow and convective mass transport increase. However, the development of turbulent flow under some conditions could lead to longer time responses, due to eddies and recirculation of substrates in the hydrodynamic boundary layers over the sensor. A biosensor that is not operating in a diffusion-limited mode may be subject to measurement errors (stirring artifact) when flow is increased.

1.4.13 Temperature Dependence

All of the physical properties, such as diffusion coefficients, gas and chemical solubilities of the liquids, and solid materials used in the construction of a biosensor will vary with temperature. The rates of enzyme-catalyzed reactions are very temperature dependent. Heat can be produced in some chemical reactions, which can change the biosensor temperature. It is common practice to restrict measurements to isothermal conditions, using either a circulating thermostatted water bath or an electrically heated metal block.

1.4.14 Signal to Noise

Electromagnetic noise, especially 60 Hz powerline interference, can be reduced by careful shielding of the biosensor and the electrical leads to the cathode and anode. Modern voltmeters have very high common mode rejection ratios. When current is measured, the major source is Johnson noise due to random electron movements in the feedback circuit. The root mean square error for Johnson noise is given by

$$E_n = \sqrt{4kR_fTf_0} \qquad (9)$$

where k is Boltzmann's constant, R_f is the amplifier feedback resistance, T is temperature in Kelvin, and f_0 is the cutoff frequency of the amplifier. Since the output voltage signal of the amplifier is $V = IR_f$, where I is the measured current, the signal-to-noise ratio can be written as

$$\frac{S}{N} = I \sqrt{\frac{R_f}{4kTf_0}} \qquad (10)$$

The S/N ratio can be reduced by reducing the cutoff frequency of the amplifier, or by passing the output through analog filters. However, important information might be missed if the bandwidth of the amplifier and output filters is limited too much. Alternately, digital filtering techniques can be used later to clean up the signal. Another technique for improving the S/N ratio of repeated signals is simple ensemble averaging. The averaging must be synchronized with the repetitive stimulus for this method.

1.4.15 Lifetime

The biological elements used in a biosensor are generally the least stable components of the system. An important property of biosensors is the length of time that they remain sensitive under normal operational conditions. The lifetime may be dependent on the total number of measurements made, or may depend on the magnitude of the analyte concentrations measured. Higher concentrations may lead to more rapid losses in sensitivity. Also, there might be other chemical species in the samples that could accelerate the deactivation process, independent from the concentration of target analyte. Another important property is the length of time that the biosensor can be stored between usage. It may be necessary to store the biosensor under refrigeration, or the biological element may need to be supplied with a specific chemical environment to maintain its bioactive properties.

1.4.16 Biocompatibility

This issue is relevant to biosensors that have medical applications where either acute monitoring or long-term implantation in the human body would be required. These biosensors might require insertion directly into the bloodstream, where blood clotting and platelet interactions must be minimized. Other devices may be inserted into tissues in various organs, where inflammatory responses and undesired growth of scar or fibrous tissues around the device could impair the biosensor performance. A substantial amount of research is being directed towards the development of biomaterials that are more biocompatible. Efforts are also being made to incorporate pharmaceutical agents directly into membranes, or to use antithrombogenic surface coatings to suppress blood clotting. Such devices would also need to be sterilized, without impairing the bioactivity of the biological element or affecting the transducer sensitivity.

1.5 IDEAL MEASUREMENT SYSTEMS

1.5.1 Direct Contact

The simplest measurement method is to have the biosensor probe directly in contact with the biological media. The biosensor must not alter the chemical environment in any way by excessive depletion of the detected species or by generation of other chemical species that might affect the sample. For fluids, the probe can simply be immersed into the sample. The ideal biosensor would not be influenced by the fluid velocity. For probes inserted into living cells and tissues, there must not be any damage to the biological sample. Biocompatibility is also imperative for long-term measurements, when the probe is left at a fixed location, as discussed previously. In other cases, important information can be derived by moving the probe through the sample. Chemical gradients or distributions of the detected chemical species within the sampled volume may be of interest.

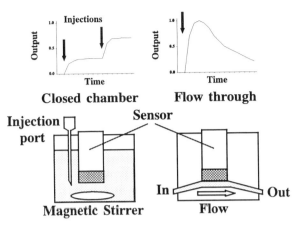

FIGURE 1.7. *Schematic drawings of two modes for making biosensor measurements. Left side: steady state responses after injecting sample into a closed, well-mixed system. Right side: transient responses following injection of sample into input stream of flow through system (flow injection analysis).*

1.5.2 Closed Chamber

If it is not possible to place the probe directly into the sample, a small volume of the fluid or any other medium (homogenized tissue, cultured cells) is removed and injected into a closed chamber. A schematic drawing for this discrete sampling method and the resulting measurement is shown on the left side of Figure 1.7. The temperature of the chamber and sample can be readily controlled by a circulating water jacket or by electrical heating. The sample might completely fill the chamber, or it could be diluted by a known amount in a larger fluid volume. In the latter case, it may be convenient to have some means for rapidly mixing the fluid within the chamber. After injecting the sample, the system is allowed to come to steady state and the resulting measurement is made. The biosensor need not have a rapid response time for these measurements, as long as the steady state response is reached after a reasonable time period.

1.5.3 Flow Injection Analysis

It may be convenient to have a flow through system in which small samples can be injected, as shown in the schematic drawing on the right side of Figure 1.7. The biosensor output signal shown in Figure 1.7 might represent an injection of analyte into the flowing stream that passes by the biosensor. The flowing stream could be either liquid or gaseous. For this sampling technique, transient measurements must be made and interpreted. The biosensors used for flow injection systems must have rapid response times to follow the time course of change. In some applications, it may be necessary to continuously monitor the biological sample. This might be accomplished by withdrawing fluid and pumping it through a temperature-regulated chamber. If it is necessary to return this fluid back to its source or to deliver it to another biosystem, the biosample should not be contaminated. It is also possible to have a system where other biological material remains at fixed sites (such as cultured cells or microbes) within the chamber, while fluid flowing over the biomaterial picks up the chemical species produced and carries it past the biosensor for detection. Other chemical species might be injected into the flow stream to provoke biochemical responses from the fixed biomaterial in the chamber.

1.5.4 Differential Measurements

Often a biosensor signal must be corrected by subtracting a baseline portion of the signal that is not directly related to the target analyte. The baseline signal may be due to the presence of a chemical species that is also used or produced by the biological element. To correct for this baseline level, another measurement can be made with a second transducer that is sensitive to the common chemical species and not sensitive to the analyte. The differential measurement approach has been successfully implemented for several types of biosensors using all of the different transducer technologies.

1.6 REFERENCES

Baumberger, J. P. 1938. "Determination of the Oxygen Dissociation Curve of Oxyhemoglobin by a New Method," *Am. J. Physiol.*, 123:10.

Beecher, H. K., R. Follansbee, A. J. Murphy and F. N. Craig. 1942. "Determination of the Oxygen Content of Small Quantities of Body Fluids by Polarographic Analysis," *J. Biol. Chem.*, 146:197–206.

Blinks, L. R. and R. K. Skow. 1938. "The Time Course of Photosynthesis as Shown by a Rapid Electrode Method of Oxygen," *Proc. Natl. Acad. Sci. USA*, 24:420–427.

Buytendijk, F. J. J. 1927. "The Use of Antimony Electrode in the Determination of pH *in Vivo*," *Arch. Ned. Physiol.*, 12:319.

Chance, B. 1991. "Optical Method," *Annu. Rev. Biophys. Biophys. Chem.*, 20:1–28.

Clark, L. C., Jr. 1956. "Monitor and Control of Blood and Tissue Oxygen Tensions," *Trans. Am. Soc. Artif. Int. Organs*, 2:41–46.

Crank, J. 1956. *The Mathematics of Diffusion*. Oxford, UK: Oxford University Press.

Danneel, H. L. 1897–1898. "Über den Durch Diffundierende Gase Hervorgerufenen Restrom," *Z. Electrochem.*, 4:227–242.

Davies, P. W. and F. Brink, Jr. 1942. "Microelectrodes for Measuring Local Oxygen Tension in Tissues," *Rev. Sci. Instrum.*, 13:524–533.

Glasstone, S. 1931. "The Limiting Current Density in the Electrodeposition of Noble Metals," *Trans. Am. Electrochem. Soc.*, 59:277–285.

Heyrovsky, J. 1922. "Electrolysis with the Dropping Mercury Electrode," *Chemicke Listy*, 16:256–304.

Michaelis, L. and W. Davidoff. 1912. "Methodisches und Sachliches dur Elektrometrischen Bestimmung der Blut-Alkalescenz," *Biochem. Z.*, 46:131–150.

Michaelis, L. and A. Kramsztyk. 1914. "Die Wasserstoffionenkonzentration der Gewebssäfte," *Biochem. Z.*, 62:180–185.

Müller, O. H. and J. P. Baumberger. 1935. "A Continuous Method for Oxygen Determination," *Trans. West. Soc. Naturalists. Eighth Annual Winter Meeting, Dec. 26–28.*

Petering, H. G. and F. Daniels. 1938. "Determination of Dissolved O_2 by Means of the Dropping-Mercury Electrode," *J. Am. Chem. Soc.*, 60:2796–2802.

Sørenson, H. A. 1909. "The Importance of Hydrogen Ion Concentration," *Biochem. Z.*, 21:31–201.

CHAPTER 2

Basic Electrochemical Principles

2.1 ELECTROCHEMICAL CELLS

The current-voltage characteristics for an electrochemical cell depend on the transport of reactants in the electrolyte (measuring medium) to the electrode surface, transfer of electrons for the oxidation and reduction of electroactive chemical species, and finally, removal of the resulting reactants (Bard and Faulkner, 1980). Overall characteristics are therefore dependent on the relative mass transport and chemical reaction kinetics of these different processes. When supplied with electrical power, current passing through the cell causes the electrolysis of an electroactive chemical species, with an integer number (n) of electrons transferred for each molecule entering the reaction. The resulting electrical charge

$$Q = It = \frac{nFm}{MW} \qquad (11)$$

is proportional to the mass (m) and molecular weight (MW) of the converted chemical species, where the Faraday constant $F = 96{,}487$ coulombs for each equivalent. The electrochemical cell usually consists of an electrode pair for which the overall chemical reaction can be divided into individual reactions for each electrode. When positive current flows out into the electrolyte, the electrode is defined as the anode. The anodic current is associated with the electrochemical oxidation of the chemical species. To complete the electrical circuit, current flows from the supporting electrolyte into the second electrode, which is defined as the cathode. The cathodic current is associated with the electrochemical reduction of the chemical species. The voltage where this oxidation-reduction process occurs is called the redox potential. The total current density (i, units A/cm²) for the reduction of one mole of substance by the cell is the sum of anodic and cathodic current densities,

$$i = i_a + i_c \qquad (12)$$

and the total current (I) is found by multiplying by the surface areas of the anode and cathode.

Usually the current at one electrode is monitored, which is called the working or indicator electrode. The other electrode is known as the reference electrode. In some electrochemical measuring systems, especially those using larger electrodes, it is convenient to have a third counter or auxiliary electrode, as shown in Figure 2.1. This is especially important when the electrical resistance of the surrounding solution (R_s) is high. Microelectrodes are much less affected by the solution resistance, and can be operated in simpler, two-electrode systems using only the working and reference electrodes. The reference can be either a hydrogen, calomel, or Ag/AgCl electrode, usually placed very close to the working electrode. When an auxiliary electrode is used, it can be placed further away in the measurement solution to complete the electrical circuit. This arrangement allows the respective cathode and anode potentials at the working and reference electrodes to be measured. The simplest method of operation is to apply a constant voltage at the redox potential of the target analyte and measure the resulting current. This approach may not always be possible, and a number of other techniques have been tried.

There are a variety of excitation waveforms that can be used to drive two- or three-electrode systems. Some of the more common waveforms are illustrated in Figure 2.2. These techniques use linear voltage ramps or square waves, or combinations of both. Cyclic voltammetry [Figure 2.2(a)] simply varies the waveform between two voltages, scanning above and below the redox potential for the target analyte. However, there are limitations with this technique, especially for larger electrodes where excessive charging currents can be generated. Microelectrodes are being used more often for electrochemical measurements since they allow much more rapid scanning rates. An alternate technique is to apply a single square wave at a specific redox potential.

A staircase of potentials [Figure 2.2(b)] is presented in normal pulse voltammetry. This technique can be useful, since the briefer times of excitation can mean reduced amounts of fouling on the electrode, or buildup of reaction products. The differential pulse methods [Figure 2.2(c) and 2.2(d)] may be useful when two chemical species are present that have redox potentials which are close together. By applying potentials above and below the indi-

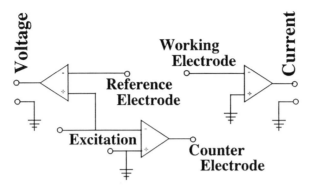

FIGURE 2.1. Schematic drawing of three-electrode configuration for electrochemical measurements. For simplicity, the resistors and capacitors required for feedback loops are not shown.

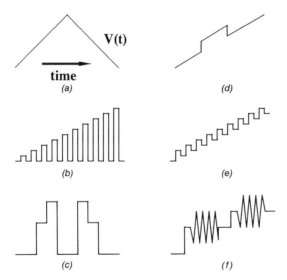

FIGURE 2.2. Common excitation signals used for electrochemical analysis: (a) cyclic, (b) normal pulse, (c) differential normal pulse, (d) differential pulse, (e) square wave, and (f) AC voltammetry.

vidual redox values, it may be possible to discriminate between the two regions. More rapid square wave or AC waveforms [Figure 2.2(e) and 2.2(f)] may have advantages for some types of electrochemical measurements. Modern electrochemical instruments are commercially available which use computers to precisely control the excitation waveforms, digitize the signals, and analyze them to determine the concentration of the target analyte.

2.2 OXIDATION-REDUCTION REACTIONS

To illustrate some principles of electrochemistry, we will consider a reversible, first order reaction in an electrochemical cell. The chemical reaction for the transformation of the oxidized chemical species C_{Ox} to the reduced species C_{Red} by the transfer of n electrons is

$$C_{Ox} + ne^- \rightleftharpoons C_{Red} \qquad (13)$$

where k_f and k_r are the first order forward and reverse rate constants respectively. Therefore, the molar rates of oxidation and reduction at the electrode surfaces

$$-\frac{dC_{Ox}}{dt} = k_f C_{Ox} - k_r C_{Red} = \frac{dC_{Red}}{dt} \qquad (14)$$

are equal but of opposite sign. The overall current density of the cell is given by

$$i = nF \frac{dC_{Red}}{dt} = -nF \frac{dC_{Ox}}{dt} \qquad (15)$$

for each mole of analyte reduced. To be completely general, chemical activities rather than concentrations should be used in the previous relationships.

The kinetics for an electrochemical reaction are complicated by the presence of an electrical field, since the forward and reverse rate constants (k_f, k_r) vary with the applied redox potential. The electrical field not only affects the electroactive species involved in the reaction, but also influences the movement of other ionic species in the electrolyte. Consequently, the activation energy required to pass through the transition state is not as well defined as it would be for ordinary first order chemical reactions. One approach has been to assume that the activation energy depends on the electrical potential (E) applied to the cell in addition to the chemical potential difference between the reactant and product.

To express the electrode currents in terms of the usual first order rate constants, a transfer coefficient (α) is usually introduced to represent the difference in energy between reactant and product as a fraction of the applied redox potential. For a single electron transfer, α is about 0.5 (Bockris and Reddy, 1970). The corresponding cathodic current is

$$i_c = nFk_f C_{Ox} \exp^{-[\alpha nFE/RT]} \tag{16}$$

and the anodic current is

$$i_a = -nFk_r C_{Red} \exp^{-[(1-\alpha)nFE/RT]} \tag{17}$$

where the universal gas constant $R = 8.314$ J/mol/K. The rate constants and concentrations in the previous equations correspond to values in the absence of an electrical field ($E = 0$).

2.3 VOLTAGE AND CURRENT AT STANDARD CONDITIONS

When the electrode reaction is at chemical equilibrium, there is no net depletion or generation of the electroactive species. Furthermore, the respective oxidant and reductant concentrations at the electrode surface and in the bulk solution must be equal. Since there is no current flow ($i = 0$) then $i_c = -i_a$, and the potential at equilibrium is

$$E_{eq} = \frac{RT}{nF} \left[\ln \left(\frac{k_f}{k_r} \right) + \ln \left(\frac{C_{Ox}}{C_{Red}} \right) \right] \tag{18}$$

Equation (18) can be written as the classical Nernst equation

$$E_{eq} = E^0 + \ln \left(\frac{C_{Ox}}{C_{Red}} \right) \tag{19}$$

where the standard electrode potential is

$$E^0 = \frac{RT}{nF} \ln (k_{eq}) \tag{20}$$

since the equilibrium constant $k_{eq} = k_f/k_r$. When the oxidant and reductant concentrations are equal ($C_{Ox} = C_{Red}$), the standard potential (E^0) and equilibrium potential (E_{eq}) are identical.

A standard first order rate constant (k^0) at the standard electrode potential (E^0) can be defined in terms of either the forward reaction

$$k^0 = k_f \exp^{-[\alpha n F E^0 / RT]} \tag{21}$$

or the reverse reaction

$$k^0 = k_r \exp^{-[(1-\alpha) n F E^0 / RT]} \tag{22}$$

when the bulk concentrations of the oxidant and reactant are equal ($C_{Ox} = C_{Red}$). A standard current exchange density

$$i_0^0 = nFk^0 \tag{23}$$

can then be defined.

Generally, the electrochemical cell is not driven at the equilibrium potential. Also, due to chemical reaction kinetics and mass transport limitations, the surface concentrations of oxidant and reductant are usually not equal to the bulk concentrations. In this case, the current densities can be expressed in terms of the overpotential

$$E_{ov} = E - E_{eq} \tag{24}$$

which is defined as the potential difference from equilibrium. The current densities, normalized with respect to the exchange current density, for the cathode

$$\frac{i_c}{i_0} = C_{Ox}^{surf} \left(\frac{C_{Red}}{C_{Ox}} \right)^{\alpha} \exp^{-[\alpha n F E_{ov} / RT]} \tag{25}$$

and the anode

$$\frac{i_a}{i_0} = -C_{Red}^{surf} \left(\frac{C_{Ox}}{C_{Red}} \right)^{1-\alpha} \exp^{-[(1-\alpha) n F E_{ov} / RT]} \tag{26}$$

are derived from the previous definitions.

When the overpotential is zero ($E = E_{eq}$), then $i_c = i_a$ and the exchange current density normalized with respect to the standard is

$$\frac{i_0}{i_0^0} = \frac{(C_{Ox})^{1-\alpha}}{(C_{Red})^{\alpha}} \tag{27}$$

which by definition must be a positive value. Reversible systems, where the chemical reaction and current exchange can occur with relative ease, will have high values for i_0/i_0^0 while irreversible systems will have low values.

2.4 STEADY STATE VOLTAMMOGRAM

The steady state relationship between current and voltage depends on the electrode geometry, rates of mass transfer of reactants and products from the electrolyte, and the chemical reaction kinetics at the electrode surface. For a planar electrode, assuming that mass transport is entirely by diffusion, the process is modeled by the one-dimensional Fick equation

$$J_i = -D_i \frac{dC_i}{dx}\bigg|_{x=0} \tag{28}$$

where the subscript i represents either the oxidized or reduced chemical species. The molar flux (J_i) to or from the electrode surface (at $x = 0$) limits the current density, which has maximum value of

$$i_{\lim} = \pm nFD_i \frac{dC_i}{dx}\bigg|_{x=0} \tag{29}$$

where the sign depends on whether the current is measured at the anode or cathode. The diffusion-limited current density must always be less than the exchange current density ($i_{\lim} < i_0$). The steady state current as a function of the overvoltage can be expressed as

$$\frac{I(E_{ov})}{I_{\lim}} = \frac{\left(1 + \frac{i_{\lim}}{i_0} \exp^{[\alpha nFE_{ov}/RT]}\right)^{-1}}{-\left(1 + \frac{i_{\lim}}{i_0} \exp^{-[(1-\alpha) nFE_{ov}/RT]}\right)^{-1}} \tag{30}$$

The resulting steady state voltammogram based on Equation (30) is shown in Figure 2.3 for $n = 1$, $\alpha = 0.5$, $T = 25°C$, and values of $i_{\lim}/i_0 = 0.0005$ (a), 0.005 (b), 0.05 (c), and 0.5 (d). Note that when $i_{\lim} \ll i_0$, there are flatter plateau regions where the currents are relatively insensitive to the overpotential.

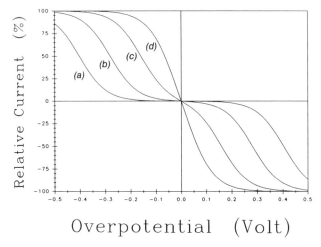

FIGURE 2.3. *Steady state voltammogram predicted from Equation (30) for n = 1, α = 0.5, T = 25°C and values of* i_{lim}/i_0 = *0.0005 (a), 0.005 (b), 0.05 (c), and 0.5 (d).*

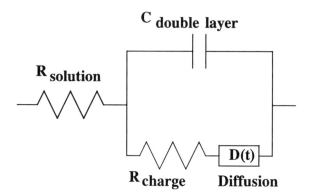

FIGURE 2.4. *Equivalent circuit for an electrochemical system.*

2.5 TRANSIENT RESPONSES

In addition to steady state operation, there are a variety of time-dependent excitation techniques that can be used to study electrochemical reaction kinetics with electrodes. Three major categories of transient techniques are: (1) potentiostatic, where the excitation voltage is changed and the resulting $I(t)$ measured; (2) galvanostatic, where the current is changed and $E(t)$ measured; and (3) coulostatic, where charge is injected to perturbate the electrode system from an initial steady state condition. For the first two techniques, various combinations of ramps and steps can be used to perturbate the system. Some of these waveforms were shown previously in Figure 2.2. For the third technique, the shape of the excitation signal does not need to be specified since only the total charge is required for the data analysis. Nagy (1990) has analyzed a number of relaxation techniques based on one-dimensional diffusion of oxidized and reduced chemical species in response to nonrepetitive electrical excitation signals. While earlier analyses were often based on step changes, he describes results for linearly rising or falling steps or pulses with finite rise times that are more often used by modern electrochemical instruments. Some of the simpler cases will be presented here.

The transient response for an electrode system is assumed to be determined by a three-step process including (1) charging or discharging of the double-layer capacity at the electrode surface, (2) oxidation-reduction reactions on the surface, and (3) diffusion of chemical reactants and products to and from the surface. An equivalent electrical circuit diagram for the electrode reaction is shown in Figure 2.4. Other equivalent circuits for electrode systems are described by Bard and Faulkner (1980). The time-dependent overpotential is modeled as a sum of charge-transfer and mass-transport terms

$$E_{ov}(t) = E_{ov}^c(t) + E_{ov}^m(t) \qquad (31)$$

which are also time dependent. The measured overpotential

$$E(t) = E_{ov}(t) + i(t)R_s \qquad (32)$$

includes an additional ohmic overpotential due to the resistance of the solution between the working and reference electrodes. The total time-dependent current density consists of a faradic term and a capacitive term, modeled by

$$i(t) = i_f(t) + C_{dl}\frac{dE_{ov}}{dt} \qquad (33)$$

where C_{dl} is the double-layer capacitance. In addition to the resistance of the solution (R_s), a resistance term for the transfer of charge can be defined as

$$R_{charge} = \frac{\nu RT}{nFi_0} \tag{34}$$

where ν is the stoichiometric number for the reaction.

Following the modeling approach described previously, Nagy (1990) obtained analytical solutions for a number of different excitation signals based on an electrode with a planar geometry. These models have been slightly redefined here by changing some of the model nomenclature. The major modification is the definition of three characteristic time scaling constants that determine the time-dependent behavior of the electrode, including the double layer,

$$\tau_{dl} = R_s C_{dl} \tag{35}$$

transfer of charge,

$$\tau_{charge} = R_{charge} C_{dl} \tag{36}$$

and the time scaling constant for diffusional transport

$$\tau_{diffusion} = \frac{\pi}{4} \left[\frac{\nu nF}{i_0 A_d} \right]^2 \tag{37}$$

where the parameter

$$A_d = \frac{1}{C_{Ox}\sqrt{D_{Ox}}} + \frac{1}{C_{Red}\sqrt{D_{Red}}} \tag{38}$$

These three characteristic time constants will be referred to again for several simple examples in the following sections.

2.6 POTENTIOSTATIC RESPONSE

Nagy (1990) describes a one-dimensional solution for the current response after a step change in voltage with amplitude E_1. With the previous modifications, his solution can be rewritten in dimensionless form as

$$\frac{I(t) - I(\infty)}{I(0) - I(\infty)} = \exp\left(\frac{t}{\tau}\right) \text{erfc}\left(\sqrt{\frac{t}{\tau}}\right) \tag{39}$$

where the instantaneous current at $t = 0$ is $I(0)$ and the steady state current is $I(\infty)$. The steady state current can either be a finite value, or it could be zero, for example in a closed system. An effective, combined characteristic time scaling constant can be defined as

$$\tau = \frac{4}{\pi}\, \tau_{\text{diffusion}} \left[1 + \frac{\tau_{dl}}{\tau_{\text{charge}}}\right]^2 \tag{40}$$

using the three characteristic time constants that were defined previously.

The normalized current change predicted by Equation (39) as a function of dimensionless time (t/τ) is shown in Figure 2.5, plotted for three different scales [(a) linear, (b) logarithmic, and (c) log-log]. The numerical values were computed using an algorithm by Miller (1981) for the complementary error function. The lowest value for Equation (39) that can be computed with this algorithm is 0.0684 for $t/\tau = 85$. The algorithm is not valid for $t/\tau > 85$. When $t/\tau = 1$, Equation (39) is equal to 0.4276. Note that this characteristic response is not linearized by any of the conventional plotting scales, except perhaps the log-log plot for the tail end of the response shown in Figure 2.5(c) (dotted line). In this case, Equation (39) is approaching an asymptotic solution, as described in the following section.

2.7 ASYMPTOTIC SOLUTIONS AND DATA TRANSFORMATIONS

At very short time, the normalized current response asymptotically approaches

$$\frac{I(t) - I(\infty)}{I(0) - I(\infty)} = 1 - \frac{2}{\sqrt{\pi}}\sqrt{\frac{t}{\tau}} \tag{41}$$

as shown in Figure 2.6(a). The short time responses are shown for Equation (39) (solid curve) and the asymptotic Equation (41) (dashed curve). When $t/\tau = 0.01$, Equation (41) underestimates Equation (39) by 1.04%. When $t/\tau = 0.05$, it is underestimated by only 0.55%.

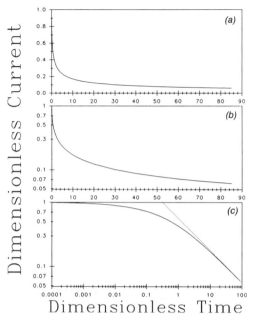

FIGURE 2.5. Dimensionless current after step change in voltage as function of dimensionless time (chronoamperometry) predicted from Equation (39) (planar electrode) for linear (a), semi-logarithmic (b), and double logarithmic (c) scaling. Asymptotic approximation at long time is also shown in Equation (42) [dotted line in (c)].

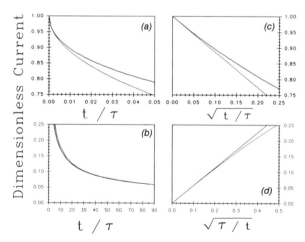

FIGURE 2.6. Short (a) and long time (b) dimensionless current predicted from Equation (39), with asymptotic solutions [dashed lines, Equations (41) and (42)]. Currents at short (c) and long time (d) are also plotted as a function of the square root of the dimensionless time ratios.

At very long time, the normalized current response asymptotically approaches

$$\frac{I(t) - I(\infty)}{I(0) - I(\infty)} = \sqrt{\frac{\tau}{\pi t}} \tag{42}$$

as shown in Figure 2.6(b). The long time responses are shown for Equation (39) (solid curve) and the asymptotic Equation (42) (dashed curve). When $t/\tau = 10$, the asymptotic solution overestimates Equation (39) by 4.90%. When $t/\tau = 50$, it is overestimated by only 0.98%. At the lowest value that can be computed using the algorithm for Equation (39) at $t/\tau = 85$, the asymptotic solution is only 0.58% higher. From Equation (42), the dimensionless times can be calculated when the electrode responses are 95, 99, and 99.9% complete ($t/\tau = 127.3$, 3,183.1, and 318,310 dimensionless time units respectively).

When the short time dimensionless current responses are plotted as a function of the square root of time as shown in Figure 2.6(c), the asymptotic solution is now a straight (dashed) line. Transformed experimental data would be nearly linear when plotted for the first 25% of the response if the planar model is applicable. When the dimensionless current responses at longer time are plotted as a function of the inverse square root of time as shown in Figure 2.6(d), the asymptotic solution is again transformed into a straight (dashed) line. Transformed experimental data would be nearly linear when plotted for the last 25% of the response, if the planar model is applicable.

An analytical solution was also obtained by Nagy (1990) for the case when the voltage step was not instantaneous. The finite rise time was modeled as a linear ramp. A series solution for the dimensionless current change is given by

$$\frac{I(t) - I(\infty)}{I(0) - I(\infty)} = \sum_{i=1}^{3} a_i \left\{ \exp\left(\frac{t}{\tau_i}\right) \operatorname{erfc}\left(\sqrt{\frac{t}{\tau_i}}\right) \right.$$

$$- \exp\left(\frac{t - t_r}{\tau_i}\right) \operatorname{erfc}\left(\sqrt{\frac{t - t_r}{\tau_i}}\right)$$

$$\left. + \frac{2}{\sqrt{\pi}} \left[\sqrt{\frac{t}{\tau_i}} - \sqrt{\frac{t - t_r}{\tau_i}} \right] \right\} \tag{43}$$

for $t > t_r$, where t_r is the rise time of the step and a_i are constants that satisfy the initial and boundary conditions for the system equations. The three effective time scaling constants $(\tau_1–\tau_3)$ can be determined from the roots of a third order equation relating the original three characteristic time scaling constants [Equations (35)–(37)].

Analytical solutions for some other common excitation waveforms can also be obtained, for example, a step pulse in voltage applied for a finite time period. The on response would be described by Equation (39). After the pulse is turned off at time t_{off}, the response would be described by a decaying exponential and complementary error function term, starting from the current reached at that time. Analytical solutions for double pulses were also obtained, which generated more complicated combinations of the exponential and complementary error function terms. Despite the relative complexity of some waveform responses, and the requirement for a numerical method to compute the complementary error function, these analytical solutions can be readily adapted to optimization procedures to determine the model parameters by curve fitting experimental data.

The chronoamperometric response has also been modeled by Bard et al. (1991). They used a numerical method to solve for the current transients generated under two different conditions of diffusion. Models for planar, microdisk, and thin-layer electrodes, with approximate solutions at short, intermediate, and long times were discussed for each case. They also showed that the geometry of the tip was very important, especially for measurements above insulating substrates.

2.8 GALVANOSTATIC RESPONSE

Following a similar modeling approach to that described in the previous section, Nagy (1990) described a one-dimensional solution for the voltage response of a planar electrode after a step change in current. The current remains on with a constant amplitude I_1. The analytical solution has been redefined here, after changing some of the model nomenclature as in the previous examples. Subtracting the potential due to the ohmic resistance of the solution $(I_1 R_s)$, the voltage response is

$$E(t) - I_1 R_s = \begin{aligned} &a_1 \left[\exp\left(\frac{t}{\tau_1}\right) \mathrm{erfc}\left(\sqrt{\frac{t}{\tau_1}}\right) + \frac{2}{\sqrt{\pi}}\sqrt{\frac{t}{\tau_1}} - 1 \right] \\ \\ &-a_2 \left[\exp\left(\frac{t}{\tau_2}\right) \mathrm{erfc}\left(\sqrt{\frac{t}{\tau_2}}\right) + \frac{2}{\sqrt{\pi}}\sqrt{\frac{t}{\tau_2}} - 1 \right] \end{aligned} \tag{44}$$

where

$$a_1 = \frac{\tau_1}{\tau_{dl} \left(\sqrt{\dfrac{\tau_2}{\tau_1}} - 1 \right)} \tag{45}$$

and

$$a_2 = \frac{\tau_2}{\tau_{dl} \left(1 - \sqrt{\dfrac{\tau_1}{\tau_2}} \right)} \tag{46}$$

The two time scaling constants

$$\tau_1 = \frac{\tau_{diff}}{2\pi^2 + 2\pi \sqrt{\pi^2 - \dfrac{\tau_{diff}}{\tau_{charge}} - \dfrac{\tau_{diff}}{\tau_{charge}}}} \tag{47}$$

and

$$\tau_2 = \frac{\tau_{diff}}{2\pi^2 - 2\pi \sqrt{\pi^2 - \dfrac{\tau_{diff}}{\tau_{charge}} - \dfrac{\tau_{diff}}{\tau_{charge}}}} \tag{48}$$

have been defined in terms of the previous characteristic time scaling constants [Equations (35)–(37)]. Note that $\tau_2 > \tau_1$. Galvanostatic responses were computed for values of $\tau_2/\tau_1 = 2$, 5, and 10, and are plotted on a linear scale as a function of the dimensionless time t/τ_1 in Figure 2.7(a).

At long time, the product of the exponential and complementary error function terms becomes small, and the normalized voltage response approaches

$$E(t) - I_1 R_s = \frac{2}{\sqrt{\pi}} \sqrt{\frac{t}{\tau_{long}}} - b \tag{49}$$

where the effective time constant

$$\tau_{long} = \left[\frac{\tau_{dl} \left(\sqrt{\tau_2} - \sqrt{\tau_1} \right)}{\tau_2 - \tau_1} \right]^2 \tag{50}$$

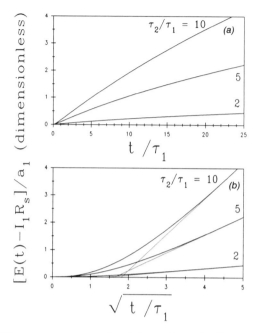

FIGURE 2.7. *Galvanostatic response for a planar electrode after a step change in current I_1 at $t = 0$ from Equation (44) (a) and transformation with $\sqrt{t}$ (b) is shown for values of $\tau_2/\tau_1 = 2$, 5 and 10 respectively. Asymptotic solutions [Equation (49)] are shown by dotted lines (b).*

and the constant

$$b = \frac{\tau_2 \sqrt{\tau_2} - \tau_1 \sqrt{\tau_1}}{\tau_{dl} \left(\sqrt{\tau_2} - \sqrt{\tau_1} \right)} \tag{51}$$

The asymptotic solutions are shown by the dotted lines in Figure 2.7(b), and are straight lines when plotted as a function of the square root of the dimensionless time.

Nagy (1990) also describes more complicated analytical solutions for double pulse excitation waveforms. These solutions have additional time-dependent exponential and complementary error function terms that appear after the second pulse. There may be some advantages in using double pulse excitation waveforms for measuring very fast reaction kinetics by precharging the double layer with the initial pulse. Of course, the frequency response of the electronic instrumentation making these types of measurements must be adequate to faithfully record very rapid events. Impedance mismatches between the amplifier, electrode leads, and the electrochemical cells are possible. Inductances in the electrode lead connections can also affect the overall response time of the measuring circuit. As a result, it is often difficult to eliminate or minimize "ringing" when step excitation signals are used.

Zoski et al. (1990) mathematically modeled galvanostatic, potentiostatic, and steady state voltammograms for hemispherical and disk-shaped microelectrodes. Their analytical solutions also contained a complementary error function and exponential function product, similar to the previous planar models. They also considered reversible and irreversible electrochemical reactions, and found similar short and long time approximations for some of the analytical solutions. They used their theory to interpret experimental current and voltage transient measurements made for the oxidation of ferrocene in acetonitrile. Two disk electrodes with diameters of 25 and 76 μm were tested. The diffusion coefficient for ferrocene was also determined from the data, and was found to be in good agreement with previous literature values. By using both galvanostatic and potentiostatic types of measurements, they showed that very fast electron transfer reactions can be studied. They also demonstrated that the same steady state voltammogram is reached by either type of measurement, although the potentiostatic data were in closer agreement with the theory than the galvanostatic data.

2.9 COULOSTATIC RESPONSE

Under ideal conditions, an instantaneous injection of current will immediately charge the double layer. Then the double layer can discharge and drive the redox reaction with no external current flowing in the circuit. If the mass transport during the relaxation is neglected, the relaxation potential after an injection of charge Q is

$$E = \frac{Q}{C_{dl}} \exp^{-t/\tau_{charge}} \qquad (52)$$

where the time scaling constant τ_{charge} was defined previously by Equation (36). Nagy (1990) describes a more complicated solution when mass transport is influencing the measurement involving differences in exponential and complementary error function expressions.

2.10 REFERENCES

Bard, A. J. and L. R. Faulkner. 1980. *Electrochemical Methods. Fundamentals and Applications*. New York, NY: J. Wiley and Sons.

Bard, A. J., G. Denault, R. A. Friesner, B. C. Dornblaser and L. S. Tuckerman. 1991. "Scanning Electrochemical Microscopy: Theory and Application of the Transient (Chronoamperometric) SECM Response," *Anal. Chem.*, 63:1282–1288.

Bockris, J. O'M. and A. K. N. Reddy. 1970. *Modern Electrochemistry*. New York, NY: Plenum Press.

Miller, A. R. 1981. *Basic Programs for Scientists and Engineers*. Berkeley, CA: Sybex Inc., pp. 277–290.

Nagy, Z. 1990. "DC Relaxation Techniques for the Investigation of Fast Electrode Reactions," in *Modern Aspects of Electrochemistry (No. 21)*, R. E. White, J. O'M. Bockris and B. E. Conway, eds., New York, NY: Plenum Press, pp. 237–292.

Zoski, C. G., A. M. Bond, E. T. Allison and K. B. Oldham. 1990. "How Long Does It Take a Microelectrode to Reach a Voltammetric Steady State?" *Anal. Chem.*, 62:37–45.

CHAPTER 3

Electrochemical Transducers in Biology and Medicine

The following types of electrochemical transducers are commonly used for a wide range of applications, and have been modified for use in biosensors, as will be discussed in later chapters. The biological and medical applications have been so extensive that only a brief review of the operational principles and some representative examples are presented here.

3.1 GLASS pH ELECTRODES

The general definition of pH, derived from Nernst steady state chemical equilibrium conditions, is

$$pH = -\log_{10}(\alpha_{H^+}) \qquad (53)$$

where α is the activity of the hydrogen ion. The glass pH electrode, shown schematically in Figure 3.1, has achieved the widest commercial use. There are several types of glass that are sensitive to hydrogen ions (H^+), and are therefore capable of a selective Nernst response. The principle of operation is proton exchange through the hydrated layers on the inside and outside of the glass, with only sodium ions moving charge within the glass itself. However, the operational pH range may be limited due to significant errors at extreme alkaline or acidic conditions. A generalized, semi-empirical form of the Nernst potential, known as the Nicolsky-Eisenman equation, can be used to describe the operation of an H^+ (pH)–sensitive glass electrode

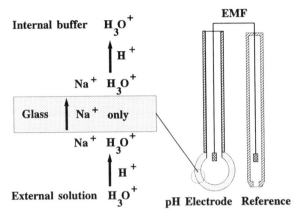

FIGURE 3.1. *Glass pH electrode. The electomotive potential (EMF) is the result of protons (H^+) exchanging through hydrated gel layers on each side of the pH-sensitive glass. Only Na^+ ions are exchanged in the glass itself.*

as the primary electroactive species (H^+) with the summation of interferences

$$E = E^0 + \frac{RT}{F} \ln \left[\alpha_{H^+} + \sum_{j=1}^{n} K_{H^+,j}(\alpha_j)^{1/z_j} \right] \qquad (54)$$

where α_j are the activities, z_j are the charges, and $K_{H^+,j}$ are the individual selectivity values for the glass to each interfering chemical species (j) in the external medium. Interfering species may include alkali metals or other ions. Sodium is usually the most significant interfering alkali metal, with much less interference from potassium.

The pH-sensitive glass is filled with an electrolyte, and must be referenced to an external calomel or Ag/AgCl electrode, as illustrated in Figure 3.1. Errors can result from liquid junction potential (E_j) effects, which are always generated when solutions with different ionic compositions come into contact. The total ionic flux depends on passive diffusion and migration due to any passage of electrical current, and also may be influenced by convective transport of the electroactive species. Based on a theory developed by Henderson (1908), a simplified equation for E_j can be written as

$$E_j = \frac{\sum_i z_i u_i (a_i - a_i')}{\sum_i z_i^2 u_i (a_i - a_i')} \frac{RT}{F} \ln \frac{\sum_i z_i^2 u_i a_i'}{\sum_i z_i^2 u_i a_i} \qquad (55)$$

where z_i is the ionic charge, u_i is the absolute mobility of the ion, a_i is the single ion activity in the sample, and a_i' is the activity in the reference electrolyte. In addition to E_j, a potential can also be generated due to contacts between different metals used in connecting the electrode. This potential would remain constant, independent of changes in the ionic composition of the measurement medium. The reference state potential (E^0) in Equation (54) therefore is the sum of the true reference potential at a given temperature, plus the sum of the junction and metal contact potentials. The reference should be stable and have a minimal liquid junction potential for accurate pH measurements.

3.2 METAL OXIDE pH ELECTRODES

Glass pH electrodes can be easily broken and are not always the best choice for some measurement conditions. A stronger and more durable pH electrode can be made from solid metals that have metal oxide surfaces.

3.2.1 Basic Theory

Generally, if a metal (M)–metal oxide (M_xO_y) reaction is reversible, it can be represented as

$$M_xO_y + 2y(e^- + H^+) \rightleftharpoons xM + yH_2O \tag{56}$$

and the equilibrium potential will increase linearly with pH. However, it is also possible to have metal oxide–metal oxide reactions where additional reversible higher and lower valency oxide couples (M_xO_y, $M_x'O_y'$) are influencing the pH potential. A metal oxide–metal oxide reaction such as

$$2MO_y + 2H^+ + 2e^- \rightleftharpoons (2y - 1)M_2O + H_2O \tag{57}$$

would have a potential change of 59 mV/pH unit at 25°C since only one H_2O molecule is involved. Combined reactions can complicate the electrode potential when more than one form of metal oxide is present.

Further complications can arise if the metal oxide becomes hydrated. For example, a reaction such as

$$MO_{[(x+n)/2]}[H_2O]_{(y+m)} + ne^- + nH^+$$

$$\rightleftharpoons MO_{(x/y)}[H_2O]_y + \left(m + \frac{n}{2}\right)H_2O \tag{58}$$

can occur. If the metal oxide is sparingly soluble, it may be possible to have steady state chemical equilibrium with adequate exchange current densities. However, if the oxide dissolves and diffuses away (corrosion), the electrochemical properties of the electrode will change with time. In this case, the electrode potential could also be sensitive to flow as convection influences the rate of oxide removal.

3.2.2 Antimony pH Electrodes

Since the early 1920s, the antimony (Sb)–antimony oxide (Sb_2O_3) electrode has been a viable alternative to the glass pH electrode, especially in highly corrosive environments (for example, in hydrogen fluoride) where glass pH electrodes do not behave well. Antimony pH electrodes can be fabricated from crystalline or powdered material, or made by plating metal from solution. Monocrystalline electrodes have been found to be more stable than polycrystalline electrodes. One of the major problems with antimony electrodes is related to the purity of the metal substrate. Instabilities can be caused by the anodic corrosion reaction and resulting surface pitting.

The reactions are usually represented by

$$2Sb + 3H_2O \rightarrow Sb_2O_3 + 6H^+ + 6e^- \tag{59}$$

at the antimony anode while O_2 is reduced

$$O_2 + 4H^+ + 4e^- \rightarrow 2H_2O \tag{60}$$

at the cathode, which can be an Ag/AgCl reference. Therefore, ambient O_2 can have a relatively large effect on the potential. The resulting equilibrium potentials for the two reactions are

$$E_{anode} = 0.15 - 2.303 \frac{RT}{nF} \text{pH} \tag{61}$$

and

$$E_{cathode} = 1.23 - 2.303 \frac{RT}{nF} \text{pH} + \frac{RT}{4nF} \ln PO_2 \tag{62}$$

The antimony electrode could be used as an O_2 sensor if the pH is maintained at a constant value. Gláb et al. (1989) have discussed the O_2 sensitivity of the antimony pH electrode, which appears to be much greater than some other metal oxide electrode types.

3.2.3 Other Metal Oxide pH Electrodes

Gláb et al. (1989) also describe some preparation methods for metal oxide pH electrodes of various types. Iridium oxide is another material that has been investigated for use in pH sensors. In addition to producing simple wire electrodes, iridium can also be sputtered onto other substrates. However, there are technical problems with producing a stable iridium oxide layer. Heating (800 to 900 °C) in a highly oxidizing flame is one method. Another popular technique uses heating in a flame after first immersing the tip in a 1 M or greater solution of either sodium or potassium hydroxide. Palladium oxide has also been used as a pH sensor. A similar technique of flame heating after treating with a strong hydroxide solution is recommended over simple heating. Apparently both iridium and palladium can form single and double oxides, which complicate their pH sensitivity, through multiple reactions such as those given by Equation (58). Iridium and palladium oxide pH sensors are reported to be insensitive to interference from ambient O_2.

3.3 pH-SENSITIVE MEMBRANES

Ammann (1986) has published a book on the use of neutral carrier ion-selective membranes for electrodes, including those for pH measurements. The main component of the membrane is a complexing ligand which is an ionophore that is specific for H^+ or other ions. These ionophores can either form channels, or physically complex with individual ions and act as carriers. The latter ionophore types have proven to be the most useful. An ionophore for H^+, tri-*n*-dodecylamine, is commercially available (Fluka Chemika, Basel, Switzerland) in formulations for use in liquid-filled pH-sensitive microelectrodes or in solid pH-sensitive polymer membranes. The ionophore may be incorporated into either polyvinyl chloride or silicone rubber membranes. After incorporation, the pH-sensitive membranes can have shelf lives up to several years when stored in the dark at normal room temperatures. The membranes are highly specific, with minimal interferences from other ions.

3.4 OXYGEN ELECTRODES

U.S. patent #2,913,386 was awarded to L. C. Clark, Jr. on Nov. 17, 1959, for his membrane-covered O_2 electrode design. A schematic drawing of the membrane-covered O_2 electrode is shown in Figure 3.2. The electrochemi-

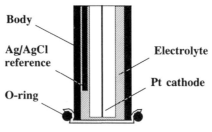

Gas permeable membrane

FIGURE 3.2. *Schematic drawing of Clark (1956)–type membrane-covered O_2 electrode. Noble metal cathode is polarized at -0.7 V relative to reference.*

cal theory, practical design considerations and construction materials, instrumentation, and many other aspects of the Clark-type membrane-covered O_2 electrode have been considered in books by Hoare (1968), Fatt (1976), Hitchman (1978), and Linek et al. (1988).

3.4.1 Cathode

The most probable electrochemical reaction at the cathode of the O_2 electrode is thought to involve two steps. O_2 is first reduced

$$O_2 + 2H_2O + 2e^- \rightarrow H_2O_2 + 2OH^- \tag{63}$$

then

$$H_2O_2 + 2e^- \rightarrow 2OH^- \tag{64}$$

where the maximum number of electrons is four.

3.4.2 Anode

The anode completes the electrical circuit. The following reaction

$$4Ag + 4Cl^- \rightarrow 4e^- + 4AgCl \tag{65}$$

is thought to occur. Since hydrogen peroxide (H_2O_2) is a stable intermediate product, the reaction kinetics can become more complicated if Equation (64) does not occur. This can happen if H_2O_2 diffuses away, or if some other chemical process (such as would occur in the presence of catalase) causes its decomposition back to O_2 and H_2O. The total stoichiometric number of electrons would decrease to two if all of the H_2O_2 escapes from the sensor. This is not thought to be a significant factor in the stagnant electrolyte-membrane-covered configuration for typical Clark-type O_2 electrode designs. However, this could become a problem for bare-tipped O_2 micro-electrodes near a source for convective transport.

3.4.3 Electrode Materials

Gold (Au) and platinum (Pt) are the most common noble metals used for the cathode. Pt may be used more frequently since it can be more easily sealed in glass. Silver (Ag) and a number of other metals and metal alloys have also been tested. Carbon cathodes can also reduce O_2, although more negative (< -1 V) potentials are usually required. Beran et al. (1978) evaluated four different O_2 electrode cathode/anode combinations, including Au or Pt cathodes with Ag/AgCl anodes, an Ag cathode and a lead (Pb/PbO$_2$) anode, and an Au cathode with a cadmium (Cd) anode. They tested a total of 10 electrodes from each group continuously for 80 hours in flowing bicarbonate buffers in a tonometer system where the PO$_2$ could be changed. All electrodes were designed as monopolar intravascular catheters, with the cathodes coated by a polyhydroxyethyl methacrylate (HEMA, or Hydron) membrane approximately 400 to 600 μm thick. The anodes were not included in the catheter assembly, and were intended for contact on the patient's skin or through an intravenous line.

The Au cathode–Ag/AgCl anode O_2 electrodes were found to stabilize more quickly than the other designs, and had the least drift. The Pt cathode–Ag/AgCl anode O_2 electrodes were nearly as good, with slightly more drift, while the other two types had much larger variations. Degradation of the anodes may have been a factor in the poor performance of the latter two designs. Aging effects on the Pt cathodes may have been due to formation of oxides on the surface. This is thought to be much less of a problem with Au cathodes, which are preferred by many researchers who use O_2 electrodes.

3.4.4 Surface Preparation

Various schemes for cleaning the cathode surface have been investigated. Mechanical abrasion using fine diamond particles or other material is often done, although it may be difficult to completely remove particles of the abrasive material afterwards. Chemical etching by chromic or nitric acid has been found to be effective in cleaning the cathode surface, but should be restricted to cathodes sealed in glass since this technique can erode most plastics. Electrochemical anodization, where a 1 to 2 V positive potential or a periodic voltage is applied for several minutes, has also been found to be effective in restoring cathode sensitivity after long use. Murphy et al. (1976) conducted aging tests with glass-sealed 50 μm diameter Pt-Ir cathodes. Typically, there was some loss in sensitivity after 8–12 hours of operation. They found that the sensitivity could be restored by anodization at +1.45 V for 30 minutes. They also found that electrodes receiving periodic anodization for a relatively short five-minute period at +1.25 V every 90 minutes improved the long-term performance. Short exposures to negative voltages (< -1.5 V) may also be effective, since this will cause H_2 gas evolution, which may lift off absorbed material on the cathode surface.

3.4.5 Membranes

A number of different membrane materials have been evaluated for use with O_2 electrodes. Besides their thickness and permeability to O_2, which are important for determining the time response of an O_2 electrode as discussed in Chapter 1, there are other factors to consider. These include the mechanical strength of the membrane and its permeability to H_2O vapor. Linek et al. (1988) summarized some of the data in the literature reporting measured properties of different membrane materials. Silicon rubber has the highest permeability for O_2, allowing around 3 to 4×10^{-14} mole O_2/m/sec/Pa when there are liquid phases on each side of the membrane. Even higher O_2 fluxes through the membrane can be achieved when there are gases on each side. Silicon rubber is also more permeable to H_2O vapor than the other membrane materials. A possible disadvantage of silicon rubber membranes is that they are a mechanically weak (flexible) material and can be easily deformed by pressure fluctuations, especially when samples are injected or flushed from the measurement chamber. This can alter the O_2 electrode sensitivity. Teflon membranes are often used since they are relatively strong. Also, they can be steam-sterilized and can tolerate higher temperatures than most of the other plastics. Teflon has the next highest O_2 permeability, about an order of magnitude less than silicon rubber, and is the material with the lowest permeability to H_2O vapor. Mylar can also be steam-sterilized and has the highest temperature tolerance. However, it has the lowest O_2 permeability, about 1,000 times smaller than silicon rubber. Polyethylene membranes are also frequently used for O_2 electrodes, and have permeabilities that are a little lower for O_2 and a little higher for H_2O vapor compared to Teflon membranes.

3.4.6 Electrolyte

Various ionic compositions have been used for the supporting electrolyte in the body of the electrode. Ferris (1983) noted that most of these formulations were proprietary information of the medical instruments industry that produced the various clinical blood gas instruments at the time. He described two formulations from his own studies based on analytical grade KCl solutions buffered with 0.1 M Tris (hydroxymethyl) aminomethane in deionized H_2O. Neutral and alkaline solutions are preferred, since they tend to extend the plateau range of the steady state voltammogram (illustrated in Figure 2.3), which is not as wide in acidic solutions. It is also desirable to have a well-buffered electrolyte, especially when the electrode is exposed to samples with different CO_2 levels, which can alter the pH. Sodium bicarbonate and sodium or potassium phosphate buffers have been commonly used. Saturated KCl solutions are regarded as less reliable by some investigators, since it is thought that chloride in the electrolyte can promote migration of Ag particles from the anode to foul the cathode surface. However, this should not be a problem when the anode is relatively far from the cathode.

Ferris (1983) found that the cause of failure for some O_2 electrodes could be traced to excessive growth of crystal "whiskers" around the anode, shorting out the electrical path. This was probably due to water evaporation from the electrolyte. O_2 and similar electrochemical transducers have been designed with variable volumes for the electrolyte reservoir. With a larger reservoir, the maintenance time between changing the electrolyte can be extended, since H_2O evaporation through the membrane has little effect on the total fluid volume. Sodium nitrate or potassium phosphate have been used to reduce evaporation by lowering the H_2O vapor pressure of the electrolyte. However, an excessively large electrolyte reservoir can cause measurement errors. The reservoir can act as a source or sink for O_2, depending on the previous history of the electrode environment. This storage effect could also change the final steady state equilibrium in a closed chamber by adding to or taking up significant amounts of O_2 from the sample. Furthermore, the electrode time response is complicated due to side diffusion effects, and large electrolyte reservoirs can cause prolonged tailing of the response. Linek et al. (1988) have done extensive mathematical modeling to take membrane, electrolyte, and mass transport boundary layer effects next to the membrane into account. They have also reviewed other theoretical models for O_2 electrodes that have appeared in the literature.

3.4.7 Body

Plastics used in the construction of the electrode body or the sample chamber may also affect the O_2 electrode measurement. Marshall et al. (1986) recognized this problem as a source of error for measurements of cell respiration with conventional Clark-type membrane-covered O_2 electrodes. They used a specially designed O_2 electrode with the body constructed entirely from ceramic and glass, and used a small electrolyte reservoir, so that minimal O_2 storage effects would occur. A U.S. patent (#5,030,336) for this modification of the Clark electrode was awarded to Cameron Koch on July 9, 1991. Stevens (1992) has recently evaluated how much O_2 is stored by seven plastics that have been used commercially for O_2 electrode systems. He equilibrated small pieces of these plastics to room air, then measured the O_2 released into a closed, liquid-filled glass chamber initially equilibrated at a hypoxic O_2 level. Nylon released the least amount of O_2, while Teflon released the most. The results for the remaining plastics, in order of increasing O_2 release, were acetal, polyvinylchloride, acrylic, high-density polyethylene, and polycarbonate.

3.5 CARBON DIOXIDE ELECTRODES

A CO_2 electrode was first developed by Stowe et al. (1957) and quickly improved by Severinghaus and Bradley (1958). The principle for electrochemical CO_2 measurements is illustrated in Figure 3.3.

3.5.1 Basic Theory

When CO_2 is dissolved in water, it can exist in two forms: as dissolved gas (PCO_2, which is equal to αCO_2 from Henry's law) and as carbonic acid (H_2CO_3). At steady state chemical equilibrium, the concentrations of CO_2

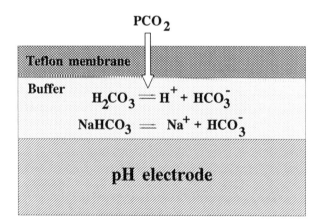

FIGURE 3.3. *Principle of carbon dioxide electrode based on pH measurement with dissociation of carbonic acid and sodium bicarbonate.*

and H_2CO_3 are equal. The partial pressure can be related to the pH of the sample since H_2CO_3 dissociates into H^+ and HCO_3^-. When another ionic buffer, such as sodium bicarbonate ($NaHCO_3$) is present, the pH is related to PCO_2 and the activity of the sodium ion by

$$pH = -\log_{10} \frac{K_1 \alpha PCO_2}{a_{Na^+}} \qquad (66)$$

where K_1 is the dissociation constant and α is the solubility coefficient for CO_2. Since the sodium ion activity remains relatively constant, the pH change is directly related to PCO_2.

3.5.2 Electrode Construction

A CO_2 gas-permeable membrane, such as Teflon or silicon rubber, is placed over a glass pH electrode or another type of pH-sensitive transducer. Sometimes a nylon mesh or another type of physical spacing element is placed between the pH transducer and the membrane to maintain a buffer reservoir near the transducer. Usually sodium bicarbonate is used as the buffer in the electrolyte.

3.6 HYDROGEN GAS ELECTRODES

3.6.1 Basic Theory

At positive polarization voltages in the range from $+0.25$ to $+0.65$ V, H_2 gas is oxidized at the anode

$$H_2 + 2OH^- \rightarrow 2H_2O + 2e^- \qquad (67)$$

Most investigators prefer to use Pt anodes, often treated with platinum black to increase the effective surface area. Substances such as ascorbate (ascorbic acid, or vitamin C), H_2O_2, and uric acid can interfere with the measurement, especially at the higher polarization voltages. Potentials at the lower range are often used to minimize these interferences, although a greater interference from O_2 can exist. Hydrogen gas diffuses more rapidly through the membrane materials that are commonly used for O_2 electrodes.

3.6.2 Applications

The polarographic measurement of H_2 has been useful as a means for estimating blood flow in different tissues, as reviewed by Young (1980). Tissue hydrogen washout curves after changing the inspired gas mixtures from a low level of H_2 (to avoid accidental explosions) to room air have been useful for this purpose, although the washout times can be rather lengthy. Another technique is to use bolus injections of H_2 gas–equilibrated solutions into the bloodstream, relating the transient tissue H_2 response to local blood flow. Electrodes have also been designed using short pulses of electrochemically generated H_2 from larger electrodes near the transducer. Again, the washout of the H_2 is related to local blood flow. The latter two methods are more rapid and can be repeated more frequently to follow temporal changes in blood flow.

There have also been biotechnology applications for H_2 electrodes. Hydrogen gas can be produced by various biochemical processes, especially by microbes living in anaerobic conditions, including the *Escherichia coli* that inhabit our own lower digestive tracts. Therefore, H_2 could be present at background trace levels for normal metabolic conditions in tissues, depending on the *Escherichia coli* activity. However, H_2 is metabolically inert and is therefore a good chemical species for washout types of measurements.

3.7 HYDROGEN PEROXIDE ELECTRODES

3.7.1 Basic Theory

In the polarization voltage range from $+0.6$ to $+0.7$ V, H_2O_2 is reduced at the anode by

$$H_2O_2 \rightarrow 2H^+ + O_2 + 2e^- \tag{68}$$

Usually Pt or Au is used for the anode, although the reaction can also take place on carbon surfaces. As with O_2 electrodes, an Ag/AgCl reference is used to complete the circuit by

$$2AgCl + 2e^- \rightarrow 2Ag + 2Cl^- \tag{69}$$

Therefore, the same basic membrane-covered electrode design used for O_2 electrodes has also been used for detecting H_2O_2. Of course, the membrane must be permeable to H_2O_2. A calibration curve for a bare, 25 μm Pt anode sealed in glass for a range of H_2O_2 concentrations from about 0.03 to 3 mM in isotonic saline was measured, as shown in Figure 3.4. The polarographic current was amplified with a Keithley 610C electrometer at $+0.65$ relative to an Ag/AgCl reference, and digitized by computer. A nonlinear relation-

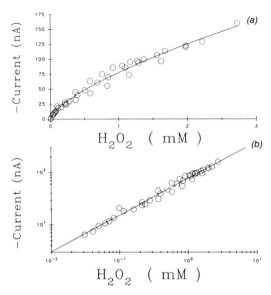

FIGURE 3.4. Nonlinear calibration curve for H_2O_2 (a) using a glass-sealed, 25 μm diameter Pt electrode polarized at +0.65 V. Calibration is linearized by a double logarithm plot (b).

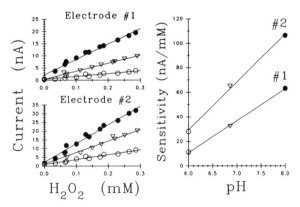

FIGURE 3.5. Example of pH dependence for H_2O_2 electrode at low concentration range (approximately linear region). Two different size Pt electrodes were calibrated (left side) in three pH buffers and the pH effect on sensitivity determined (right side).

51

ship was observed over this range [Figure 3.4(a)]. A double logarithmic plot [Figure 3.4(b)] linearized these data. The current in nanoamperes for this electrode was given by $I = 77.7 \times [H_2O_2]^{0.687}$ where the H_2O_2 concentration is in mM.

The author has investigated the pH sensitivity for bare Pt H_2O_2 electrodes by changing H_2O_2 concentrations in three phosphate buffers with pH values at 6.0, 6.84, and 8.0. Results for two Pt electrodes are shown in Figure 3.5. Both electrodes were made from glass-sealed 25 μm Pt wires. Electrode #1 was ground at a perpendicular angle, while the second electrode was ground at a more oblique angle and had a little larger surface area. As shown in the two panels on the left side of Figure 3.5, the currents for each electrode were approximately linear at the lower concentration range < 0.3 mM, but were strongly pH dependent. The sensitivity was reduced in the more acidic conditions, and was greater with more basic pH, as shown in the panel on the right of Figure 3.5.

Several electroactive chemical species, including ascorbate, uric acid, and acetaminophen have been reported to interfere with the H_2O_2 electrode, since they are reduced within the same potential range. It may be possible to reduce these higher molecular weight interferences by placing an appropriate membrane over the electrode. As discussed further in Chapter 4, this type of electrode has been very useful for monitoring some types of enzyme-catalyzed reactions where H_2O_2 is a product. H_2O_2 is not normally a background chemical species under normal metabolic conditions.

3.8 CARBON SURFACE ELECTRODES

Various carbon-based electrodes have been constructed from materials including glassy carbon, reticulated vitreous carbon, graphite/epoxy composites, pyrolytic graphite, carbon pastes, carbon powders, and carbon fibers. Electrochemical reactions for carbon-based electrodes have been rather intensely investigated during the past two decades, with special attention to increasing sensitivity with chemically modified surfaces. Electrocatalysts for highly specific reactions can be attached by the free valences that are available on the carbon surface. Attachment can be achieved by simple adsorption or through reactions that promote chemical binding. Functional catalysts can also be immobilized in membranes, polymers, or gels over the carbon surface. Carbon-based electrodes that have been used for some *in vivo* bioelectrochemical measurements may be less prone to surface fouling by proteins that might occur with more conventional noble metal electrodes. However, as often occurs with other types of bioelectrodes, carbon electrode properties are usually altered after prolonged use in tissues or exposure to biological fluids. Inactivation of surface catalysts, interference from other oxidized or reduced chemical species, poor signal-to-noise ratios, and other problems that affect long-term stability need additional study and further refinements.

Ormonde and O'Neill (1990) have studied some mechanisms that might be responsible for the reduced sensitivity of carbon paste electrodes after exposure to tissue. Teflon tubes (320 μm O.D., 250 μm I.D.) were filled with a carbon powder/silicone oil paste to form a disk-shaped electrode. Only the electrode sensitivity to ascorbic acid was investigated. After testing, some electrodes were implanted in rat brain for several hours, then were removed and retested. Other electrodes were exposed to a surfactant (Triton-X), lipid (phosphatidylethanolamine), or bovine serum albumin. Electrode resistance and double-layer capacitance were determined using cyclic voltammetry at 50 mV/sec. Differences between potentials for the anodic and cathodic peaks were measured, and changes in the rates of electron transfer and adsorption were calculated.

Ormonde and O'Neill found that the surfactant reduced the carbon paste electrode resistance from an average of 156 kOhm to 3 kOhm, suggesting that the silicone oil at the surface is responsible for most of the electrode resistance. The thickness of the paste had no effect on the reduction in resistance after exposure to surfactant. The carbon paste electrode capacitance increased from 37 to 500 nF after exposure to surfactant. Lipid exposure had similar effects, reducing resistance to 16 kOhm and increasing capacitance to 290 nF. Tissue exposure caused the largest changes, reducing resistance to 2 kOhm and increasing capacitance to 830 nF. The position of the ascorbic acid oxidation wave was shifted to a lower potential with either surfactant, lipid, or tissue exposure. Sensitivity to ascorbic acid also declined for each treatment or with exposure to albumin.

Ormonde and O'Neill concluded that removal of oil from the electrode surface allows faster electron transfer from ascorbic acid, while adsorption of lipids and proteins block a portion of the active sites. They also suggested that lipophilic substances like stearic acid should not be used, since they will not remain effective in increasing sensitivity to dopamine due to the removal of hydrophobic elements after implanting electrodes in brain tissue.

3.9 ION-SENSITIVE ELECTRODES

Presently, there are about 30 cations and anions that can be detected by various types of ionic sensors. Both solid and liquid membranes have been developed in a variety of configurations. In addition to pH-sensitive glass, other types of glass can be used for ionic measurements, again using the Nernst equilibrium principle. However, glass electrodes tend to be slow and relatively difficult to miniaturize. More recent success has been achieved with several types of ion-sensitive membranes, which have mobile sites for ion exchange.

3.9.1 Basic Theory

The generalized Nicolsky-Eisenman relationship [Equation (54)], including the summation of interfering species, can also be used to describe the operation of an ion-sensitive electrode as

$$E = E^0 + \frac{RT}{z_a F} \ln \left[\alpha_a + \sum_{j=1}^{n} K_{a,j} (\alpha_j)^{z_a / z_j} \right] \qquad (70)$$

where the activity of the primary electroactive species is α_a with valence z_a; and α_j are the activities, z_j are the valences, and $K_{a,j}$ are the individual selectivities (relative to the analyte) for the ion-sensitive membrane to each interfering chemical species (j) in the external medium. A recent book by Ammann (1986) describes natural and synthetic ionic carriers, their theory of operation, and a general survey of different ion-sensitive electrodes. Another recent book by Coşofreţ and Buck (1992) includes an appendix that summarizes some of the major characteristics for commercially available membrane sensors for ammonium, bromide, calcium, chloride, copper, fluoride, iodide, lead, potassium, silver, and sulfide ions from a dozen different companies.

An example of a calibration curve obtained by the author with a K^+ microelectrode he fabricated using a neutral carrier ionophore (cocktail B, Fluka Chemical, Switzerland) is shown in Figure 3.6. The electrode was back-filled with 100 mM KCl. Further fabrication details are discussed in Chapter 5 for ion-sensitive and other types of microelectrodes. The voltage (EMF) for the microelectrode was measured with a Keithley model 614 electrometer and digitized by computer. The sensitivity was tested by sequentially diluting or adding concentrated KCl solutions, starting from 100 mM. A semi-logarithmic relationship was found, as expected from theory [Equation (70) with no interfering species], with a sensitivity around 95 mV per decade of KCl concentration, as shown by the regression line in Figure 3.6.

3.10 OTHER ELECTROCHEMICAL DETECTION METHODS

Modern electrochemical scanning techniques have been used for the direct detection of other important analytes, such as glucose and urea.

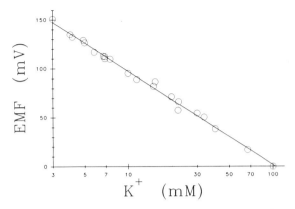

FIGURE 3.6. *Typical semi-logarithmic voltammetric calibration for a K$^+$-sensitive microelectrode using a neutral carrier ionophore.*

However, there still are many difficulties with using direct electrochemical techniques for measurements in blood under *in vivo* conditions.

3.10.1 Glucose

Yao (1991) has reviewed some electrochemical methods for detecting glucose using cyclic voltammetry. Cyclic measurements in the range from -1 to $+1$ V were obtained in physiological buffer solutions, and oxidation peaks were found at -0.72 V during the anodic scan and around -0.8 V in the cathodic scan. Another method investigated was by compensated net charge cyclic voltammetry, which involves integration of the current over one potential cycle. Reduced interferences from other chemical species were reported using this method.

Bindra and Wilson (1989) applied membranes made from Nafion alone, or with collagen over an Au working electrode. The membranes improved the pulsed amperometric detection of glucose in a flow injection apparatus. The Nafion-coated Au electrode was 2.4 times more sensitive than a bare Au electrode. A modified electrode with collagen over the Nafion was about 1.3 times more sensitive. After allowing a several hour period of stabilization for the initially high background current, a detection limit of about 25 nM glucose was found. A linear response based on the area under the peak response curves was found for measurements in both aqueous phosphate buffers and in human blood serum with different glucose concentrations. The interference from urea and ascorbate was found to be significantly reduced by the Nafion membrane, to only about 5% at maximum anticipated physiological concentrations. Bare electrodes had much larger interferences, around 140% for example with 2 mg/dL ascorbate. Acetaminophen interference was also reduced, although high concentrations could still cause some problems. Potential interferences from amino acids were also investigated. Bare Au electrodes were found to be practically insensitive to glucose in physiological concentrations of amino acids. Some effects were found with the Nafion-treated electrodes, but they remained sensitive to glucose. Bindra and Wilson (1989) suggested that some of the measurement errors could be partially compensated for by calibrating electrodes in standard glucose solutions containing the interferences at anticipated physiological background levels.

3.10.2 Urea

Patzer et al. (1991) report another cyclic technique for direct electrochemical detection of urea, which is oxidized in the $+0.5$ to $+1.1$ V range. In this case, an external timed relay switch was used to reverse the polarity of two Pt electrodes in a cyclic fashion. During one part of the cycle, one of the Pt electrodes was subjected to a step increase in current while monitoring the voltage. A galvanostatic response would be measured, similar to that shown previously in Figure 2.7 for Equation (44). When an upper voltage limit of 1.1 V was reached, the relay switched off the current, applying it to the second electrode. Hence, a continuous measurement can be made by sequentially monitoring the two electrodes. However, each electrode oxidizes urea over only half of the cycle, allowing time for the surface to recover. Some experimentation was required to find an optimum duty cycle. If switched too frequently, the urea conversion rate would be too low since there would not be sufficient time to reach the oxidation potential. If the cycling rate was too slow, the electrode would be at a higher potential and would not efficiently oxidize urea. Glucose is also oxidized during part of the cycle, and the relative amount of current used to oxidize glucose and urea can be calculated for each. Unfortunately, a very large component of unknown origin was also included in the measurement. Also, if this technique were to be used in blood, other species would likely cause considerable interferences with the measurement.

3.10.3 Nitrogen Gas Transducer

Although dissolved N_2 is not directly oxidizable or reducible, Robblee and Brunelle (1991) were able to develop an electrochemical sensor for measuring N_2. A sensor in a 15 gauge hypodermic needle was made, with a metal cation (M^{+n}) surface coated by a hydrophobic gas-permeable membrane. The principle of operation is based on the formation of a stable metal-N_2 complex from the reaction.

$$M^{+n-1} + N_2 \xrightarrow{k'} M^{+n-1}-N_2 \tag{71}$$

where the metal cation is activated by applying a potential to generate the reducing species (M^{+n-1}). A first order rate constant (k') was found from a plot of M^{+n-1} with time. The sensor is restored to its original state by applying an oxidizing potential ramp to regenerate the metal cation. The sensor was tested at pressures ranging from 1 to 10 atmospheres, and a linear relationship was found for the sensor output as a function of the N_2 partial pressure. Reproducibility was ±5% in room air saturated solution, and within ±0.5 to 2% at higher atmospheric pressures. Measurements could be repeated every three to five minutes, and could be made more rapidly at the higher N_2 pressures.

3.11 CLINICAL APPLICATIONS OF ELECTROCHEMICAL TRANSDUCERS

3.11.1 Blood Chemistry

The application of the Clark-type O_2 electrode and CO_2 electrodes for the measurement of human blood PO_2 and PCO_2 by discrete sampling techniques was an immediate success. Radiometer (Copenhagen, Denmark) introduced the first automated blood gas analyzer (model ABL 1) in 1973. Modern clinical blood gas instruments now use microprocessors for automatic operation and self-calibration, and the electrodes are relatively easy to maintain. In addition to O_2, CO_2, and pH, clinical instruments are also available for measurements of blood Na^+, Ca^{2+}, and K^+ and other physiologically important ions from discrete blood samples. These instruments are vital to clinical laboratories in hospitals throughout the world. Other electrochemical techniques for clinical blood and urine measurements are also under development, as reviewed by Meyerhoff (1990).

A disposable, flow through electrochemical system for bedside monitoring of the bloodstream is commercially available (GEM-6, Mallinckrodt Sensor Systems). The sensor cartridge has electrochemical transducers to measure Na^+, Ca^{2+}, K^+, pH, PCO_2, and PO_2. An electrical conductivity method is used to measure hematocrit. The blood sample must be periodically withdrawn from indwelling catheters placed in the patient. There continues to be a great interest in extending O_2 electrode technology to both invasive and noninvasive devices to make continuous measurements of blood and tissue O_2 levels, as reviewed by Kreuzer and Kimmich (1984), and more recently by Mendelson (1991).

3.11.2 Catheter Electrodes

Intravascular PO_2 and PCO_2 catheters would be very useful for monitoring the blood gas status during many surgical procedures, or for general long-term monitoring of patients undergoing intensive care. The catheter must be small enough to enter a 4F (1.33 mm) diameter opening for placement into a femoral, brachial, or radial artery. A potential source of interference for O_2 electrodes can come from volatile halogenated anesthetics, as Severinghaus et al. (1971) first noted for halothane. Albery et al. (1978) found that nitrous oxide (NO_2) was also reduced by the O_2 electrode. Electrodes polarized at a more negative potential (-900 mV instead of -650 mV) were found to have more interference from NO_2. Albery et al. (1987) exploited the increased interference at -900 mV to monitor the level of NO_2 anesthesia in blood. A number of membrane modifications, including the use of Mylar membranes, have been investigated over the years to reduce interference from volatile anesthetics.

It is also possible to measure other physiological variables with catheter systems using electrochemical transducers. For example, Collison et al. (1989) describe a combination K^+ and PCO_2 catheter, which has been tested in human blood *in vitro*, but has not yet been used for intravascular measurements in humans. Potassium may be an important variable to monitor clinically, especially in patients receiving digitalis therapy. There have also been extensive research efforts to improve the thrombogenicity of the various membrane materials used for catheters.

3.11.3 Tissue Surface Electrodes

Severinghaus (1981) modified combined PO_2 and PCO_2 transducers for transcutaneous measurements, which were subject to drift caused by interactions due to OH^- production, causing progressively more alkaline conditions in the electrolyte. He added an aluminum anode, where the reaction

$$Al + 3OH^- \rightarrow Al(OH)_3 + 3e^- \qquad (72)$$

consumed OH^-. Alternately, the following reaction

$$4OH^- \rightarrow O_2 + 2H_2O + 4e^- \qquad (73)$$

could take place at a Pt anode. Either method could be used to force the stoichiometric consumption of OH^- as it was produced. In the second method, the O_2 electrode must be placed far enough away so that the measurement is not affected by the O_2 evolved.

Transcutaneous PO_2 and PCO_2 transducers have achieved widespread use in the pediatric setting, especially for monitoring the blood gas status of neonates. This essentially noninvasive device heats the skin and causes vasodilation and maximum blood flow in the underlying blood vessels. The resulting surface PO_2 and PCO_2 measurements are proportional to the arterial blood PO_2 and PCO_2. However, these proportionality factors become more variable with age, and efforts to extend transcutaneous PO_2 and PCO_2 measurements to other applications have not been as widespread. The transcutaneous electrode may be useful in diagnosing peripheral vascular disease, where low blood flow could reduce PO_2 and elevate PCO_2 in the skin due to the compromised circulation. The device could also be employed on the surface of an organ, using a more invasive approach. The reestablishment of blood flow to grafted skin or to transplanted organs might also be evaluated with similar electrodes.

Kwan and Fatt (1970) used an unheated Clark O_2 electrode to monitor the surface PO_2 on the palpebral conjunctiva of the eye. This can be accomplished relatively noninvasively by inserting electrodes shaped like a contact lens under the eyelids. Since this tissue is receiving its blood supply from the internal carotid artery, PO_2 changes monitored in the eye may reflect changes in blood flow to the brain as well. Kram (1985) has reviewed the clinical use of polarographic O_2 electrodes and other techniques to assess tissue perfusion.

3.12 REFERENCES

Albery, W. J., W. N. Brooks, S. P. Gibson and C. E. W. Hahn. 1978. "An Electrode for pN_2O and pO_2," *J. Appl. Physiol.*, 45:637–643.

Ammann, D. 1986. *Ion-Selective Micro-Electrodes. Principles, Design and Application.* New York, NY: Springer-Verlag.

Beran, A. V., G. Y. Shigezawa, D. A. Whiteside, H. N. Yeung and R. F. Huxtable. 1978. "*In vitro* Evaluations of Monopolar Intravascular Oxygen Sensors," *J. Appl. Physiol.*, 44:969–973.

Bindra, D. S. and G. S. Wilson. 1989. "Pulsed Amperometric Detection of Glucose in Biological Fluids at a Surface-Modified Gold Electrode," *Anal. Chem.*, 61:2566–2570.

Clark, L. C., Jr. 1956. "Monitor and Control of Blood and Tissue Oxygen Tensions," *Trans. Am. Soc. Artif. Int. Organs*, 2:41–46.

Collison, M. E., G. V. Aebli, J. Petty and M. E. Meyerhoff. 1989. "Potentiometric Combination Ion/Carbon Dioxide Sensors for *in vitro* and *in vivo* Blood Measurements," *Anal. Chem.*, 61:2365–2372.

Coşofreţ, V. V. and R. P. Buck. 1992. *Pharmaceutical Applications of Membrane Sensors*. Boca Raton, FL: C.R.C. Press.

Fatt, I. 1976. *Polarographic Oxygen Sensors*. Cleveland, OH: C.R.C. Press.

Ferris, C. D. 1983. "Design and Fabrication of Polarographic Oxygen Sensors," *J. Clin. Eng.*, 8:201–211.

Gláb, S., A. Hulanicki, G. Edwall and F. Ingman. 1989. "Metal–Metal Oxide and Metal Oxide Electrodes as pH Sensors," *Anal. Chem.*, 21:29–47.

Henderson, L. J. 1908. "Concerning the Relationship between the Strength of Acids and Their Capacity to Preserve Neutrality," *Am. J. Physiol.*, 21:173–179.

Hitchman, M. L. 1978. *Measurement of Dissolved Oxygen*. New York, NY: J. Wiley and Sons.

Hoare, J. P. 1968. *The Electrochemisty of Oxygen*. New York, NY: Wiley Interscience.

Kram, H. B. 1985. "Noninvasive Tissue Oxygen Monitoring in Surgical and Critical Care Medicine," *Surg. Clin. N. America*, 65:1005–1024.

Kreuzer, F. and H. P. Kimmich. 1984. "Techniques Using O_2 Electrodes in Respiratory Physiology," in *Techniques in Respiratory Physiology—Part I*, A. B. Otis, ed., Ireland: Elsevier, pp. 1–29.

Kwan, M. and I. Fatt. 1970. "A Noninvasive Method of Continuous Arterial Oxygen Tension Estimation from Measured Palpebral Conjunctival Oxygen Tension," *Anesthes.*, 35:309–314.

Linek, V., V. Vacek, J. Sinkule and P. Benes. 1988. *Measurement of Oxygen by Membrane-Covered Probes*. Chichester, Great Britain: Ellis Horwood Ltd.

Marshall, R. S., C. J. Koch and A. M. Rauth. 1986. "Measurement of Low Levels of Oxygen and Their Effect on Respiration in Cell Suspensions Maintained in an Open System," *Radiation Res.*, 108:91–101.

Mendelson, Y. 1991. "Invasive and Noninvasive Blood Gas Monitoring," in *Bioinstrumentation and Biosensors*, D. L. Wise, ed., New York, NY: M. Dekker, Inc., pp. 249–279.

Meyerhoff, M. E. 1990. "New *in vitro* Analytical Approaches for Clinical Chemistry Measurements in Critical Care," *Clin. Chem.*, 36:1567–1572.

Murphy, V. G., R. E. Barr and A. H. Hahn. 1976. "Control of Electrode Aging by a Periodic Anodization Technique," in *Oxygen Transport to Tissue—II*, J. Grote, D. Reneau and G. Thews, eds., New York, NY: Plenum Press; *Adv. Exp. Med. & Biol.*, 75:69–75.

Ormonde, D. E. and R. D. O'Neill. 1990. "The Oxidation of Ascorbic Acid at Carbon Paste Electrodes. Modified Response Following Contact with Surfactant, Lipid and Brain Tissue," *J. Electroanal. Chem.*, 279:109–121.

Patzer, J. F., II., S. J. Yao and S. K. Wolfson, Jr. 1991. "Voltage Polarity Relay—Optimal Control of Electrochemical Urea Oxidation," *IEEE Trans. Biomed. Eng.*, 38:1157–1161.

Robblee, L. S. and M. B. Brunelle. 1991. "An Electrochemical Sensor for Quantification of Tissue PN_2," *J. Undersea and Hyperbaric Med. Soc.*, 18(supplement):63, abstract.

Severinghaus, J. W. 1981. "A Combined Transcutaneous PO_2-PCO_2 Electrode with Electrochemical HCO_3^- Stabilization," *J. Appl. Physiol.*, 51:1027–1032.

Severinghaus, J. W. and A. F. Bradley. 1958. "Electrodes for Blood PO_2 and PCO_2 Determination," *J. Appl. Physiol.*, 13:515–520.

Severinghaus, J. W., R. B. Weiskopf, M. Nishimura and A. F. Bradley. 1971. "Oxygen Electrode Errors due to Polarographic Reduction of Halothane," *J. Appl. Physiol.*, 31:640–642.

Stevens, E. D. 1991. "Use of Plastic Materials in Oxygen-Measuring Systems," *J. Appl. Physiol.*, 72:801–804.

Stowe, R. W., R. F. Baer and B. F. Randall. 1975. "Rapid Measurement of the Tension of Carbon Dioxide in Blood," *Arch. Phys. Med.*, 38:646–650.

Yao, S. J. 1991. "Chemistry and Potential Methods for *in vivo* Glucose Sensing," in *Bioinstrumentation and Biosensors*, D. L. Wise, ed., New York, NY: M. Dekker, Inc., pp. 229–248.

Young, W. 1980. "H_2 Clearance Measurement of Blood Flow: A Review of Technique and Polarographic Principles," *Stroke*, 11:552–564.

CHAPTER 4

Enzyme-Based
Electrochemical Biosensors

4.1 ENZYME BIOCATALYSIS THEORY

4.1.1 Basic Theory

Perhaps the simplest scheme for describing a biochemical reaction catalyzed by a single enzyme E is the irreversible conversion of a substrate S to a product P

$$E + S \underset{k_r}{\overset{k_f}{\rightleftharpoons}} ES \overset{k_f^*}{\rightarrow} E + P \tag{74}$$

through the reversible formation of an intermediate enzyme-substrate complex ES. If the kinetics obey the Michaelis-Menten model, the reaction rate V is related to concentration by

$$V = -\frac{dC_s}{dt} = \frac{dC_P}{dt} = \frac{V_{max} C_s}{K_m + C_s} \tag{75}$$

where V_{max} is the maximum possible chemical reaction rate. The Michaelis-Menten constant K_m is related to the three equilibrium constants by

$$K_m = k_r + \frac{k_f^*}{k_f} \tag{76}$$

and is also defined as the concentration where the reaction rate is reduced to half of the maximum rate. One International Unit (1 U) of the enzyme is

63

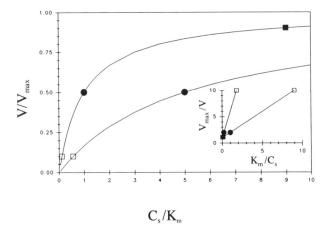

$$C_s/K_m$$

FIGURE 4.1. *Concentration-dependent reaction rate predicted from the Michaelis-Menten kinetic model. The rate is normalized by the maximum possible rate, and is plotted as a function of the concentration normalized by the Michaelis-Menten constant K_m (upper curve). The relative rate is also shown for another reaction (lower curve) with $5\times$ higher K_m. Linear Lineweaver-Burk data transformations are shown in inset for these two examples.*

defined as the amount that catalyzes 1 μM of the product per minute at a specified temperature and pH or for other relevant factors at a reference state.

4.1.2 Data Transformations

Normalized reaction rates for the Michaelis-Menten model are shown in Figure 4.1 for two different K_ms, with one K_m that is five times higher (lower curve) than the other reaction (upper curve). The 50% rate is indicated by solid circles, with values at 10% (open squares) and 90% of maximum (solid squares) also indicated for both examples. The inset in Figure 4.1 shows a Lineweaver-Burk transformation (double reciprocal plot)

$$\frac{V_{max}}{V} = 1 + \frac{K_m}{C_s} \tag{77}$$

using the points indicated on the two curves. The Eadie-Hofstee transformation

$$\frac{V}{V_{max}} = 1 - \frac{K_m}{C_s}\left(\frac{V}{V_{max}}\right) \tag{78}$$

is another popular plot that is similar, except that V/V_{max} is plotted on the *y*-axis. Both of these transformations have been derived by inverting Equation (74), and are expressed in a normalized form. Experimental data plotted by either transformation will fall along a straight line with slope K_m, and V_{max} can be determined from the *y*-axis intercept. Both transformations are only useful for characterizing biochemical reactions that follow single enzyme Michaelis-Menten kinetics.

4.1.3 Time-Dependent Measurements

It may be useful to measure the time course of substrate utilization after adding an initial concentration of analyte C_0. Assuming a closed system with no new substrate being supplied, the fall in concentration with time $C(t)$ must be found by numerical methods due to the nonlinear kinetics [Equation (74)]. Approximate solutions can also be derived, ignoring for the moment diffusional transport limitations that may exist for any of the chemical species involved. At very high substrate concentrations, the rate is approximately constant

$$\frac{dC_s}{dt} = -V_{max} \tag{79}$$

(zero order reaction) and the substrate concentration falls linearly

$$C_s(t) = C_0 - V_{max}t \tag{80}$$

with time from the initial concentration C_0. At very low substrate concentrations, the reaction is approximately first order

$$\frac{dC_s}{dt} = -\frac{V_{max}}{K_m} C_s \tag{81}$$

(i.e., linearly dependent on concentration). The time rate of change in substrate concentration approaches

$$C_s(t) = C_1 \exp^{-(V_{max}/K_m)t} \tag{82}$$

where C_1 is the substrate concentration level below which the kinetics are pseudo–first order. Both of the above approximations can be modified to follow the time-dependent change in product concentration by changing signs in Equations (79) and (81).

The approximate time-dependent solutions for analyte utilization are il-

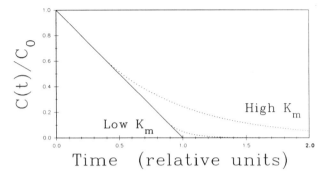

FIGURE 4.2. *Approximate time course of substrate utilization with single enzyme Michaelis-Menten reaction kinetics for high and low K_m values. The reaction begins with a zero order rate (straight line) then follows first order rates (dotted lines).*

lustrated in Figure 4.2 for two reactions that are following Michaelis-Menten kinetics with a fivefold difference in the individual K_m values. The approximate increase in product concentration would follow mirror images of these curves. If the reaction begins with a high analyte level ($C_0 \gg K_m$), V_{max} can be estimated from the initial linear slope (solid line). When K_m is very low, the utilization rate will be essentially constant for most of the analyte concentration range. It may be very difficult to estimate K_m from the tail end of the curve if K_m is very low. When K_m is high, the utilization is concentration dependent over a much wider range. The first order approximation (dotted lines) may be more useful for estimating K_m from an experimental measurement in the latter case.

An integrated form of the Michaelis-Menten kinetic model

$$\frac{V_{max}}{K_m} = \frac{1}{t}\left(\frac{C_0 - C_s}{K_m} - \ln\frac{C_0}{C_s}\right) \tag{83}$$

is also useful for examining kinetic data that have been normalized after dividing by the time. Plotting the logarithm term ($\ln C_0/C_s$)/t versus the concentration difference ($C_0 - C_s$)/t produces a linear plot with slope $-1/K_m$ and intercept V_{max}/K_m from the transformed data. Of course, to obtain the most accurate parameter estimates for V_{max} and K_m from actual biosensor measurements, it would be necessary to solve the problem numerically in concert with a least squares optimization method.

4.1.4 Inhibiting Reactions

It is also possible to inhibit enzyme-catalyzed reactions, either by competitive or noncompetitive interactions. If the inhibitor is just as likely to occupy the enzyme site, the reaction is competitive, and can be represented by

$$\frac{V}{V_{\max}} = \frac{C_s}{C_s + K_{m,s}\left(1 + \frac{C_i}{K_{m,i}}\right)} \tag{84}$$

while a noncompetitive reaction can be represented by

$$\frac{V}{V_{\max}} = \frac{C_s}{\left(C_s + K_{m,s}\right)\left(1 + \frac{C_i}{K_{m,i}}\right)} \tag{85}$$

where the inhibitor concentration is C_i and the respective Michaelis-Menten constants are $K_{m,i}$ for the inhibitor and $K_{m,s}$ for the analyte.

4.1.5 Multienzyme Systems

Many other types of biochemical reaction kinetics are possible besides the single enzyme Michaelis-Menten kinetic model, including reactions catalyzed by multiple enzyme systems. The reaction kinetics can become much more complicated than outlined above. For example, a two-enzyme system with equally random possibilities for a second enzyme catalyzing the reaction with substrate C_b can be represented by

$$\frac{V}{V_{\max}} = \frac{C_s C_b}{C_s C_b + (K_{m,s}K_{m,b} + K_{m,b}C_s + K_{m,s}C_b)} \tag{86}$$

where $K_{m,b}$ represents the Michaelis-Menten constant for the second substrate. The apparent K_m for the overall reaction would be between the values for $K_{m,s}$ and $K_{m,b}$. This can be extended to an nth order system, giving the multiplied product

$$\frac{V}{V_{\max}} = \prod_{i=1}^{n} \frac{C_i}{C_i + K_{m,i}} \tag{87}$$

where C_i and $K_{m,i}$ are the individual concentration and Michaelis-Menten constants for the interacting enzymatic pathways. The author has suggested that this type of model is appropriate for describing the apparent adaptation of oxidative metabolism with the shifts in NADH, ATP, ADP, and P_i that occur during sustained hypoxic conditions (Buerk, 1990).

Another possibility is for parallel enzymatic pathways that utilize the same substrate, given by

$$\frac{V}{V_{max}} = \sum_{i=1}^{n} f_i \frac{C_s}{C_s + K_{m,i}} \tag{88}$$

where the summation of the fractional components must equal one. The author has found experimental evidence for a two-oxidase pathway for O_2 metabolism from stop flow O_2 disappearance measurements with O_2 microelectrodes in the cat carotid body (Buerk et al. 1989a, 1989b). The carotid body serves a chemosensory role in regulating blood O_2, CO_2, and pH. The second pathway appears to have a much higher K_m for O_2 than cytochrome a,a_3, and might play a role in the control of neural firing with chemosensory stimuli in this tiny organ. Multiple pathways for O_2 also exist in other tissues. In a recent review paper, Vanderkooi et al. (1991) listed 29 oxidases known to be present in various mammalian tissues, all of which have lower affinities (higher K_ms) for O_2 than cytochrome a,a_3.

It is also possible to have secondary enzymes that catalyze biochemical reactions which amplify the primary enzyme-catalyzed reaction of interest. Secondary enzymes can be useful by recycling other substrates that enter the primary reaction. Specific examples will be examined in this and later chapters.

4.2 IMMOBILIZATION TECHNIQUES

4.2.1 Basic Theory

The purpose of immobilization is to insure that the enzyme diffusivity D_E is either zero or else much less than the diffusivities for the substrate and product, so that the enzyme activity is maintained. The effective (or apparent) reaction rate, which will be designated as app V_{max} in the following equations, depends on the concentration and activity of the enzyme. In linear Cartesian coordinates, the partial differential equations for one-dimensional diffusion which govern movement can be written as

$$\frac{\partial C_s}{\partial t} = D_s \frac{\partial^2 C_s}{\partial x^2} - \text{app} V_{max} \frac{C_s}{K_m + C_s} \tag{89}$$

for the substrate, and

$$\frac{\partial C_p}{\partial t} = D_p \frac{\partial^2 C_p}{\partial x^2} + \mathrm{app}\, V_{\max} \frac{C_s}{K_m + C_s} \tag{90}$$

for the product. If more than one substrate or more than one product is involved, additional coupled diffusion equations would be required for each chemical species.

4.2.2 Flow Injection

For flow injection systems where multiple chemical species are flowing by a biosensor, convective terms must be added to the previous equations for each species. If an analyte has been injected into a flowing stream, the general shape of the concentration change with time as it flows past the biosensor (washout curve) would need to be determined. The mathematical complexity of the resulting coupled sets of partial differential equations requires that they be solved numerically by computer. Even steady state problems require numerical procedures, although simplifications can lead to analytical solutions for certain boundary conditions. In many practical applications, less rigorous approaches have been taken which allow biosensor measurements to be interpreted on a more empirical basis.

4.2.3 Enzyme Activity

Biosensors are usually designed with high enzyme loading to insure that sufficient biocatalyst activity is available, and the enzyme is provided with an appropriate environment to sustain its activity. The local chemical and thermal environment can have profound effects on the enzyme stability. Most enzymes are unable to withstand temperatures above 50 °C. It may be necessary to keep the enzyme and the biosensor refrigerated before they are used, or between periods of use. The pH is especially critical for enzyme-catalyzed reactions, but it may not always be possible to operate at the optimum pH for a specific biochemical reaction. A number of inhibitory chemical species can be present in the biological sample, which can lead to enzyme inactivation. Impurities such as trace amounts of heavy metals can inactivate enzymes. Often ethylenediaminetetraacetic acid (EDTA) is added to the supporting electrolyte solution around the biosensor to form complexes with any heavy metal ions. Unfortunately, EDTA can also inactivate enzymes. Even under the best of conditions, there will be some natural degradation of enzyme activity with time. The ability to maintain enzyme activity, as we shall see, remains a difficult problem. A great deal of research is being directed towards the development of enzyme-based biosensors with extended shelf life and improved length of useful measurement times.

4.2.4 Immobilization Materials

As chemical substrates are utilized and products are formed, all of the chemical species must be able to move freely through the various components of a biosensor system. The biosensor would not have a very useful lifetime if the enzyme can also diffuse away. There are basically five methods for immobilizing enzymes: physical entrapment, microencapsulation, adsorption, covalent cross-linking, and covalent binding.

By physical entrapment methods, the enzymes are held in place by viscous aqueous solutions adjacent to the biosensor elements and are physically restricted by membranes to keep them from diffusing away. The outer membranes must be permeable to the chosen analyte. Common membrane materials have included cellophane, cellulose acetate or nitrate, poly(vinyl alcohol), and polyurethane. Some of the more common types of entrapment gels include agarose, gelatin, polyacrylamide, and poly(*N*-methylpyrrolidone).

Microencapsulation methods (for example, inside liposomes or absorbed on glass beads or fine carbon particles) can be used to physically include the encapsulated enzyme either within the membrane, or within viscous gels or porous materials near the transducer element in the biosensor. Most mem-

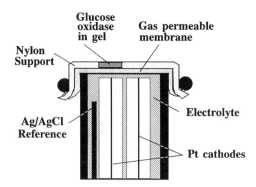

FIGURE 4.3. *Differential biosensor to measure glucose designed by Updike and Hicks (1967), using two O_2 electrodes. One electrode is used to measure ambient O_2 levels to interpret measurement for O_2 utilized in glucose oxidase–catalyzed reaction [Equation (91)] in substrate over second O_2 electrode.*

brane materials will adsorb enzymes directly on the surface, although the strength of the attachment may not always be adequate. Enzyme attachment may be strengthened by first adsorbing other proteins, for example, albumin. Silanized surfaces can also adsorb enzymes better.

Cross-linking agents, such as glutaraldehyde or glyoxal, can significantly increase the attachment. However, these agents can also interfere with the enzyme activity, especially at higher concentrations. An appropriate balance must be determined from empirical tests. If the enzyme can be covalently linked to the electrochemical transducer, it may be possible to have direct exchange of electrons. A number of different materials are being investigated, which will be discussed later in this chapter. Some of the specific applications of enzyme-based electrochemical biosensors are discussed in the following sections.

4.3 GLUCOSE BIOSENSOR

4.3.1 Basic Theory

The enzyme glucose oxidase [EC 1.1.3.4] catalyzes the oxidation of D-glucose according to the following reaction

glucose oxidase

$$\text{D-glucose} + O_2 + H_2O \rightarrow H_2O_2 + \text{D-gluconic acid} \qquad (91)$$

If either the glucose or O_2 concentration is too low, the reaction can become rate limited. Three means are available for measuring glucose concentration with electrochemical transducers: (1) the fall in O_2 as the reaction proceeds, (2) the production of H_2O_2, and (3) the change in pH with production of D-gluconic acid. The glucose biosensor has been extensively investigated with many different approaches taken to optimize sensitivity and stability.

4.3.2 Modified O_2 Electrodes

Clark and Lyons (1962) were the first to suggest the use of an electrochemical transducer (the Clark-type membrane-covered O_2 electrode) as the transducer to measure glucose concentration based on the change in O_2 in the glucose oxidase–catalyzed reaction. Updike and Hicks (1967) designed and tested the first quantitative biosensor for glucose. They used a differential design, shown schematically in Figure 4.3, with two membrane-covered Clark electrodes to measure O_2. Over one cathode, glucose oxidase was immobilized in a 25 to 50 μm thick layer of acrylamide gel supported in a nylon mesh. This cathode measured the steady state O_2 tension in the gel after some O_2 was consumed in the reaction with glucose. However, the amperometric signal from this cathode alone was not always sufficient to determine the sample glucose concentration, since the O_2 tension in the test solution might not be known. An identical thickness of gel was placed over the second cathode after heating to inactivate the enzyme. The second cathode permitted measurements of the O_2 tension in the test solution. The difference in the amperometric signals between the two cathodes was found to be linearly proportional to glucose concentration, independent of O_2 tension, within a reasonable operational range. The signal from the second cathode also provided information about conditions where the reaction might become rate limited by inadequate O_2 availability, causing the glucose biosensor measurement to become unreliable.

Gough et al. (1985) attempted to eliminate the rate-limiting behavior of the glucose oxidase–catalyzed reaction at low O_2 by designing a biosensor that oxygenated the immobilized enzyme layer. A cylindrical probe was made, with a highly O_2 permeable silicon membrane with large surface area around the outer radius. This permitted O_2 to diffuse from the solution around the biosensor and maintain a constant O_2 supply for the reaction. The surface area for the glucose-permeable membrane, placed only at the tip of the probe, was much smaller. Consequently, this probe design restricted glucose flux into the cylindrical layer of immobilized enzyme while maximizing O_2 flux. This improved, but did not eliminate, the nonlinearity of the glucose biosensor at low O_2.

4.3.3 Modified H_2O_2 Electrodes

Clark (1973) and Guilbault (1973) were the first to exploit the production of H_2O_2 by the glucose oxidase–catalyzed reaction using a Pt electrode polarized at a positive potential to electrochemically reduce H_2O_2. Of course, the reaction is still rate limited at low O_2. The amperometric signal from H_2O_2 was found to be directly proportional to glucose under steady state conditions. Also, Guilbault (1973) found that the initial rate of current change (dI/dt) could be related to glucose concentration, since it was related to the amount of H_2O_2 generated in the reaction with glucose. At the present time, the H_2O_2 electrode is probably the most widely used transducer for commercial glucose analyzers. For example, the glucose analyzer by Yellow Springs Instruments (model 23) uses a membrane-covered Clark-type electrode for detecting H_2O_2 from the glucose oxidase–catalyzed reaction. This benchtop instrument is probably the most widely used commercial biosensor, with both clinical and general laboratory applications.

4.4 BLOOD GLUCOSE MONITORING

One of the most important applications of the glucose biosensor is the monitoring of blood glucose levels in diabetics. As defined by the National Diabetes Data Group of the National Institutes of Health, a person is diagnosed as diabetic when his/her fasting blood glucose level is greater than or equal to 140 mg/dL. Normally, fasting blood glucose levels are below 115 mg/dL and the peak response to an oral glucose tolerance test would not exceed 200 mg/dL, falling below 140 mg/dL two hours later. The diabetic will have a peak response exceeding 200 mg/dL, and his/her blood glucose will remain above this level after two hours. One of the major medical advances of this century has been the development of insulin to regulate glucose metabolism. The insulin dose for an individual must be adjusted to minimize hyperglycemia while avoiding serious hypoglycemia. This requires frequent and accurate testing to monitor the diabetic's blood glucose levels.

4.4.1 Home Monitors

It is now possible for diabetics to determine their blood glucose at home. Usually this is done four times daily, before each meal and before bedtime. A drop of blood is obtained by pricking a finger. The blood sample is placed on a reagent strip, which is then analyzed by an instrument using reflectance photometry. This optical method is inherently nonlinear and requires somewhat more complicated signal analysis than other methods.

In addition, there are several problems associated with reflectance photometry. First, the instrument drifts from the factory setting and requires periodic recalibration. This places the responsibility on the user to assure that the instrument remains accurate. Some newer instruments have been designed to include an optical scanner for reading bar code information from the reagent strip which is then used to automatically recalibrate the instrument. Second, the reading is sensitive to erythrocytes and other blood elements. Glucose levels are overestimated at low hematocrit and underestimated at high hematocrit. Plasma proteins can also interfere with the reagent strip chemistry. In fact, calibration solutions for a given standard actually contain lower glucose levels, to compensate for the significantly higher reading obtained in the absence of protein. Finally, the reagent strip method is sensitive to blotting and wiping techniques, and to differences in timing when preparing and reading the sample.

In spite of these problems, the reagent strip method is relatively simple to use and has been successfully implemented. Eighteen different commercial instruments using this technology have been described by McCall and Mulling (1986).

4.4.2 Portable Monitors

Recently Updike et al. (1988) developed and tested a reusable pocket-portable blood glucose monitor that uses an electrochemical biosensor. The key feature that is crucial to the instrument design is a flexible and durable multilayered membrane containing immobilized glucose oxidase. The instrument is simple to use, operated by only one button, with instructions shown on a liquid crystal display. The instrument prompts the user to supply either a calibration solution or a drop of blood into a small plastic well. The sample can be as small as 7 μL. The plastic well holds the sample over an H_2O_2 electrochemical sensor, which is covered with the enzyme-activated membrane. The biosensor is linear with glucose concentration in the range from 0 to 500 mg/dL.

Since the current required for the electrochemical biosensor is much less than that required by light-emitting diodes used in reagent strip photometric instruments, the instrument is battery operated. Simpler electronics are required, allowing the instrument to be miniaturized to the size of a hand-held calculator. The instrument detects when the sample has been applied, and automatically times the analysis, which is completed in 30 seconds. After making the measurement, the liquid crystal display prompts the user to wipe out the blood sample and place a drop of cleaning solution into the well. A tight plastic cover is then closed to prevent evaporation or spillage, keeping the membrane hydrated until the instrument is used again. The user is then prompted to turn the instrument off, or the device automatically shuts off if inactive for three minutes.

Updike et al. (1988) subjected eight instruments, chosen at random from the first mass production run (Markwell Medical, Racine, WI), to a rigorous series of tests. Four glucose levels ranging from 57 to 347 mg/dL were prepared by adding known amounts of anhydrous D-glucose to either human plasma or heparinized whole blood. Concentrations were independently verified by Garber et al. (1979) by comparison with a standard clinical laboratory method. Replicate tests for each instrument were performed over an eight-hour period with the plasma samples. Average coefficients of variation for each instrument ranged from 2.0 to 5.0% of the true value, with an overall mean of 3.7%. Measurements for the lowest glucose concentration had the greatest inaccuracy, with average variations ranging from 2.7 to 10.5%, while the highest glucose level had the least variation, ranging from 1.9 to 4.8%.

The effects of hematocrit on the measurement up to 65% were tested by centrifuging whole blood samples and remixing with plasma. Three different glucose levels were tested and no significant interaction with hematocrit was seen. Furthermore, no interferences were found from tests with uric acid, ascorbic acid, creatinine, heparin, high lipid levels, or bilirubin. The biosensor and membrane lifetime was also evaluated, with good accuracy found after 500 measurements. Some instruments were tested for up to six weeks before a degradation in performance was seen. The sensitivity of the instrument can be restored simply by replacing the enzyme-activated membrane.

The only limitation of the blood glucose biosensor was found with measurements taken when the blood PO_2 was low (< 35 Torr), as anticipated from the rate-limited reaction [Equation (91)]. At the highest blood glucose levels, the instrument underestimated the true level by approximately 10% when the PO_2 was low. When the blood PO_2 was > 70 Torr, there was no detectable error due to O_2 limitation. For most practical applications, the O_2 sensitivity of the glucose biosensor should not be a serious problem. The pocket-portable blood glucose monitor developed by Updike et al. (1988) has a relatively low cost and is easier to operate than some other commercial instruments.

4.4.3 Implantable Glucose Biosensors

Ideally, a closed loop system for regulating the delivery of insulin could be developed, using an implanted glucose biosensor for precise feedback control based on biological demand. A more tightly regulated control of insulin during the early stages of the disease may spare the diabetic from more severe microcirculatory complications later in life. Shirichi et al. (1986) tested a needle-type glucose biosensor for controlling insulin delivery to diabetic patients. The biosensors had to be changed every four days, and clinical tests were limited to only a week. Despite considerable research efforts, summarized in reviews by Wilkins (1989) and Pickup (1989), at the present time there is no reliable glucose biosensor available for long-term patient monitoring. Invasive devices that are in direct contact with blood are very difficult to maintain and are risky for routine patient use. Devices implanted in tissues tend to measure lower glucose levels than in the bloodstream, and may have significant time delays, lagging behind the blood glucose levels. Even if these problems can be solved, the natural degradation of glucose oxidase in the biosensor remains a significant limitation. Consequently, most programmable insulin delivery systems are open loop systems that are not feedback controlled.

Xie and Wilkins (1991) recently described a potential solution to this problem, using an enzyme rechargeable design. Glucose oxidase was immobilized on a very fine (<325 mesh), ultrapure carbon powder using albumin and 2.5% glutaraldehyde for cross-linking. Lampblack and graphite powders were also tested. The operational lifetime, for a fall in sensitivity to 30% of the initial value, was nearly three months for the ultrapure carbon powder and about two months for the graphite powder. The poorest lifetime, only a couple of weeks, was found with lampblack. The body of the biosensor was designed so that the old volume of carbon particles and enzyme could be easily removed and a fresh volume injected to revitalize the biosensor. This design might be clinically useful for subcutaneously implanted glucose biosensors, which could be easily accessible for repeated refilling without requiring additional surgery.

4.5 INDUSTRIAL GLUCOSE MONITORING

Industrial applications for glucose biosensors include monitoring fermentation broths or food processing procedures where glucose is a key ingredient that must be kept within certain ranges. Batch processes where cultures of microbes or cells must continually receive adequate nourishment have also been monitored with glucose biosensors. Other sugars such as fructose, lactose, maltose, and sucrose are also of interest for some industrial processes. Successful methods for detecting other carbohydrates have been developed, usually based on splitting the molecule with enzymes to produce glucose, which can then be detected by a glucose biosensor (Guilbault et al., 1991). For example, to detect sucrose, invertase has been used, adding mutarotase to help convert glucose from its α- to β-anomer. Other enzymes that break down carbohydrates to glucose, such as galactosidase to break down lactose and glucoamylase to break down maltose, have also been used. Biosensors based on the previous modified glucose biosensors may have applications for industrial process monitoring. In addition, many other types of biosensors have found industrial applications as reviewed by Arnold and Meyerhoff (1988), including biosensors for amino acids, alcohols, and sulfites.

4.6 UREA BIOSENSOR

4.6.1 Basic Theory

The enzyme urease [EC 3.5.1.5] catalyzes the hydrolysis of urea

$$\text{urease}$$

$$(NH_2)_2CO + 2H_2O + H^+ \rightarrow 2NH_4^+ + HCO_3^- \tag{92}$$

to produce ammonium ion NH_4^+ and bicarbonate. The first potentiometric urea electrode was developed by Guilbault and Montalvo (1969), using an ion-selective electrode to follow NH_4^+. This appears to be the most useful approach. However, pH changes and CO_2 changes can also be monitored. Nilsson et al. (1973) used urease immobilized on a glass pH electrode for a urea sensor based on pH changes. Guilbault and Shu (1972) have investigated a urea sensor based on CO_2 measurements.

4.6.2 Applications

The reliable detection of urea also has potential medical applications, particularly for portable hemodialysis systems for treating patients with renal disease either at home or in the hospital. Urea, uric acid, creatinine, and methylguanidine can accumulate in the bloodstream of patients with renal disease, eventually reaching toxic levels if they are not removed. One commercial blood analysis instrument (NOVA 12, Nova Biomedical, Waltham, MA) has both glucose and urea biosensors as part of its multianalyte detection capability using discrete blood samples.

4.7 ALCOHOL BIOSENSORS

4.7.1 Basic Theory

Alcohol sensors have been developed using alcohol oxidase [EC 1.1.3.13], which catalyzes the reaction

$$\text{alcohol oxidase}$$

$$\text{alcohol} + O_2 \rightarrow H_2O_2 + \text{acetaldehyde} \qquad (93)$$

The reaction can be monitored with either an O_2 electrode or H_2O_2 electrode. However, earlier systems using alcohol oxidase were not very successful due to low enzyme activity and short lifetimes.

4.7.2 Applications

Guilbault et al. (1983) found that coimmobilizing alcohol oxidase from *Candida boidinii* with catalase increased the enzyme lifetime for several months. Only an O_2 electrode could be used as the sensing element, since catalase would influence the measurements from an H_2O_2 electrode. Lubrano et al. (1991) used a newly developed, stable, and more active alcohol oxidase from *Pichia pastoris* (Provesta Corporation, Bartlesville, OK). Alcohol biosensors using either O_2 or H_2O_2 transducers were evaluated.

Several different membrane/enzyme sandwich arrangements were tested using polycarbonate membranes (Nucleopore Corp., Pleasanton, CA) or a combined silicon rubber/polycarbonate membrane (General Electric, Schenectady, NY). The polycarbonate membrane is hydrophobic and has small (0.03 μm) pores that allow ethanol to diffuse freely across the membrane. Alcohol oxidase was mixed with different glutaraldehyde mixtures to immobilize the enzyme, then pipetted onto the dull side of the polycarbonate membrane and allowed to dry in air for two hours. The activated membrane was then soaked in a phosphate-buffered saline solution. Different combinations of glutaraldehyde (ranging from 0.18 to 2%) and increasing amounts of alcohol oxidase (ranging from 1 to 20 units) were investigated. Both the current and the rate of current change in response to ethanol concentrations up to 0.5% were measured for three different membrane arrangements. All of the various combinations of membranes were arranged with the alcohol oxidase in the center. One type had polycarbonate membranes both on the outside and on the inside covering an H_2O_2 sensor. Another had a polycarbonate membrane on the outside, with a membrane-covered O_2 electrode on the inside.

The sandwich arrangement for the H_2O_2 electrode, and the O_2 electrode arrangement was found to be linear only to about 0.02% ethanol, then the steady state current reached a plateau. The best results were obtained with the silicon rubber/polycarbonate membrane on the outside and a polycarbonate membrane on the inside, covering an H_2O_2 electrode. With this arrangement, the H_2O_2 current was linear up to 0.5% ethanol concentration, with a lower detection limit of 0.0002% ethanol.

Lubrano et al. (1991) also performed tests on other alcohols and other possible interfering substrates. The alcohol oxidase sensor was also found to be very sensitive to methanol. The response for a low concentration of methanol (0.32 mg/dL) was 117% relative to the response to a concentration of 22 mg/dL ethanol. The sensor was also sensitive to n-propanol, where a response of 28.7% for a 0.58 mg/dL concentration was measured. The response to isopropanol at 8.1 mg/dL was only 8.09% relative to ethanol. Ascorbic acid, a major interfering chemical species for H_2O_2 electrodes, was only 0.01% at a concentration of 1,640 mg/dL. The other substances tested for possible interference included acetaminophen, acetylsalicylic acid, caffeine, d-mannose, d-fructose, d-galactose, cholesterol, cholic acid, uric acid, and tyrosine. There were either no measurable interferences or else they were negligibly small (<0.01%). The effect of pH (5 to 9.8 pH range) on steady state currents and maximum initial rates was also investigated for the sensor response to 0.02% ethanol. Relatively small pH dependencies of 5.2% and 2.7% per pH unit were found respectively. Some of this reduction in pH dependence of the H_2O_2 sensor can be attributed to the phosphate buffer in the middle layer. However, some of the other membrane sandwich designs had much greater pH dependencies, suggesting that the external sample was able to diffuse into the middle layer and change its pH. This could not only directly affect the sensitivity of the H_2O_2 sensor, but could also shift the enzyme activity of the alcohol oxidase away from its optimal activity.

Another operational principle for alcohol sensors is based on the presence of the enzyme alcohol dehydrogenase (ADH), which catalyzes the oxidation reaction for primary alcohols, given by

$$\text{ADH}$$

$$\text{alcohol} + \text{NAD}^+ \rightarrow \text{aldehyde} + \text{NADH} + \text{H}^+ \qquad (94)$$

while secondary and tertiary alcohols are not affected. As described further in Chapter 6, the chemiluminescence of NADH can also be monitored by fiberoptic biosensors.

4.8 MORE SINGLE ENZYME BIOSENSORS

There are a large number of single enzyme biosensors that can be coupled to conventional O_2, H_2O_2, and pH electrodes or other types of ion-sensitive transducers for analyte measurements. Clark (1973) listed 24 other oxidoreductases besides glucose oxidase which produce H_2O_2 and presented some preliminary results for an amino acid biosensor using the H_2O_2 electrode as a transducer. As mentioned earlier in this chapter, Vanderkooi et al. (1991) listed 29 oxidases known to be present in various mammalian tissues. The specific analytes involved in the bioreactions catalyzed by these oxidases could be detected in biosensors with O_2 electrode transducers. Tables listing specific biosensors have been compiled by Bardeletti et al. (1991), Coulet et al. (1991), Kauffman and Guilbault (1991), Macholán (1991), and others. For example, one of the tables published by Macholán (1991) lists over 100 chemical species that can be detected by biocatalytic membrane biosensors. Grouped in general categories, these include alcohols and aldehydes, amines, amino acids, carbohydrates, lipids, nucleic bases, phenols, and other chemical species. Some representative examples are discussed as follows.

4.8.1 Lactate Biosensor

Leland Clark received a U.S. patent (#4,467,811, August 28, 1984) for a lactate biosensor based on the reaction

$$\text{L-lactate} + O_2 \xrightarrow{\text{lactate oxidase}} \text{pyruvate} + H_2O_2 \tag{95}$$

and using either an O_2 or an H_2O_2 electrode as the transducer. Lactate is produced in tissues when O_2 is not available. The clinical monitoring of blood lactate (lactic acid) levels would be useful for quantifying the severity of myocardial infarction or as an indicator of heart failure, and for assessing the severity of shock or the progression of some diseases. Reliable blood lactate measurements would also be of interest in sports medicine. A blood lactate catheter biosensor has been designed and patented by Shun Lim (U.S. patent #4,830,011, May 16, 1989). Waite et al. (1991) described preliminary results for this catheter, which uses an H_2O_2 electrode with a commercially available lactate oxidase membrane (Yellow Springs Instruments, Inc.). Nine catheters were fabricated and tested in physiological saline buffers with lactate concentrations of 5, 10, or 15 mM. Response times (10 to 90% change) averaged about 75 seconds. The average nonlinearity of the catheters was 5.88% full scale, with a 2.48% standard deviation.

4.8.2 Biosensors Using pH Electrodes

Kumaran et al. (1991) tested several types of single enzyme biosensors using a glass pH electrode as the transducer. A very thin 1 to 2 μm coat of gelatin (0.01% w/v) derived from porcine skin was applied to the pH electrode. Four enzymes were tested: acetylcholinesterase [EC 3.1.1.7], butyrylcholinesterase [EC 3.1.1.8], penicillinase [EC 3.5.2.6], and urease [EC 3.5.1.5]. After the first gelatin coating had dried, the pH electrode was dipped into one of the enzyme solutions for 20 minutes. The enzyme-coated electrode was allowed to dry, then it was sprayed for three seconds with 2.5% glutaraldehyde by an airbrush while rotating the pH electrode at 50 r.p.m. The acetylcholinesterase biosensor had the best lifetime, lasting 10 to 14 days before a progressive drop in sensitivity was observed. The biosensors were stored wet at 4°C overnight between tests.

4.8.3 Biosensors Using Ammonia Transducers

Ammonia can be detected, as indicated previously for the urea biosensor, using either indirect pH changes or directly with NH_4^+ ion-sensitive membranes. Biosensors for amino acids can utilize NH_4^+ transducers, through a reaction such as

arginine deaminase

$$\text{L-arginine} \rightarrow \text{citrulline} + NH_3 \qquad (96)$$

or by using other enzymes that act on amino acids. Alanine, asparagine, aspartate, aspartame, glutamine, histidine, methionine, and tryptophan have been detected using NH_4^+ ion-sensitive transducers with the specific enzymes.

4.8.4 Biosensors Using PCO_2 Transducers

Some amino acids can also be degraded to form CO_2, such as the reaction

tyrosine decarboxylase

$$\text{tyrosine} \rightarrow \text{tyramine} + CO_2 \qquad (97)$$

catalyzed by tyrosine decarboxylase. Histidine and lysine can also be detected by a PCO_2 transducer using decarboxylases specific for these amino acids.

4.9 MULTIPLE ENZYME BIOSENSORS

It is possible to combine several enzymes to achieve sensitivities for analytes where a single enzyme may not be adequate, or to convert the product of one reaction to another chemical species that can be more readily measured by conventional transducers. In addition to some of the entries listed in the tables of specific biosensors mentioned in the previous section, examples of multienzyme biosensors can also be found in reviews by Arnold and Meyerhoff (1988), Janata and Bezegh (1988), and others. Biosensors have also been designed with enhanced sensitivities by using a second enzyme system to recycle key substrates. A few examples for multienzyme biosensors are described as follows.

4.9.1 Free Fatty Acids

Sode et al. (1989) designed a biosensor for fatty acids based on the following two-step process. In the first step, acyl coenzyme-A synthetase catalyzes the reaction

$$\text{acyl-CoA synthetase}$$

$$R-CH_2CH_2COOH + R'CO-CoA \rightarrow$$

$$R-CH_2CH_2CO-CoA + R'COOH$$

$$\text{ATP} \rightarrow \text{AMP} \tag{98}$$

$$Mg^{++}$$

where acyl coenzyme-A is added to the fatty acid in the presence of ATP and Mg^{++}. In the second step, acyl coenzyme-A oxidase catalyzes the formation of a double bond

$$\text{acyl-CoA oxidase}$$

$$R-CH_2CH_2CO-CoA + O_2 \rightarrow RCH{=}CHCO-CoA + H_2O_2 \tag{99}$$

using O_2 in the process. Sode et al. (1989) used a photo-cross-linkable poly(vinyl alcohol) polymer to entrap enzymes on a cellulose nitrate membrane, which was then placed over the Teflon membrane of a Clark-type membrane O_2 sensor. They tested aqueous emulsions of oleic and palmitic fatty acids. The biosensor was linear from 0.38 to 2 mM for oleic acid, and was linear to 2.6 mM for palmitic acid. This two-enzyme biosensor was simpler to make and much more sensitive than a five-enzyme, sequential bioreaction type of biosensor that had been tested previously by the same research group. Besides clinical applications for measuring free fatty acids in blood, a fatty acid biosensor might also have applications in the food industry to measure the early stages of denaturation in oily foods.

4.9.2 Fish Freshness Biosensor

One of the more elaborate biosensor designs has been developed to test fish freshness by Wantanabe and Tanaka (1991) from the Tokyo University of Fisheries. In order to understand the principles on which the biosensor system is based, consider the following sequence of reactions

$$\text{ATPase}$$

$$\text{ATP} \rightarrow \text{ADP} + P_i$$

$$\text{myokinase}$$

$$\text{ADP} \rightarrow \text{AMP} + P_i$$

$$\text{AMP deaminase}$$

$$\text{AMP} \rightarrow \text{IMP} + NH_3$$

$$\text{5-nucleotidase}$$

$$\text{IMP} \rightarrow \text{inosine} + P_i$$

$$\text{nucleoside phosphorylase}$$

$$\text{inosine} \rightarrow \text{ribose-1-phosphate} + \text{hypoxanthine}$$

$$\text{xanthine oxidase}$$

$$\text{hypoxanthine} + O_2 \rightarrow \text{xanthine}$$

$$\text{xanthine oxidase}$$

$$\text{xanthine} + O_2 \rightarrow \text{uric acid}$$

(100)

which detail seven successive steps in the breakdown of adenosine triphosphate (ATP) to uric acid as tissue undergoes enzymatic autolysis and eventual spoilage. The depletion of high-energy phosphates (ATP, ADP, AMP) and accumulation of inosine and hypoxanthine alters the taste and quality of the meat.

The chemical species for the last stages of this process were monitored, using four enzyme-modified O_2 electrodes. A sample of fish meat was homogenized and sampled by a flow injection technique. The first biosensor was modified using only xanthine oxidase, and would detect either hypoxanthine or xanthine, consuming O_2 as indicated for the last two steps in Equation (100). The second biosensor was modified using both xanthine oxidase and nucleoside phosphorylase, and would therefore be sensitive to ino-sine, as well as hypoxanthine and xanthine. The third biosensor used xan-thine oxidase, nucleoside phosphorylase and 5-nucleoside phosphorylase, and was therefore sensitive to inosine-5-monophosphate (IMP), inosine, hypoxanthine, and xanthine. The fourth biosensor was modified with four enzymes: xanthine oxidase, nucleoside phosphorylase, 5-nucleoside phosphorylase, and AMP deaminase, and was therefore sensitive to adenosine-5-monophosphate (AMP), inosine-5-monophosphate (IMP), inosine (INO), hypoxanthine (HX), and xanthine. Signals from the four biosensors were measured and digitized by computer. An algorithm was devised to interpret the enzyme-catalyzed reactions and interactions among the four biosensors. A fish freshness factor, defined as

$$K = \frac{INO + HX}{ATP + ADP + AMP + IMP + INO + HX + \text{uric acid}} \times 100\%$$

(101)

was the final computed result, allowing fish to be classified as very fresh when $K < 10\%$, fresh when $K < 40\%$, or not fresh when $K > 40\%$.

4.9.3 Amplification by Enzyme Recycling

Macholán (1991) has reviewed research using additional enzyme-catalyzed reactions to amplify the response that a biosensor would achieve from a primary reaction catalyzed by a single enzyme. This concept is based on recycling a substrate through the second reaction, which then reenters the primary reaction. The net effect is to generate more of the reaction product that is detected by the transducer. This allows much lower detection limits for the analyte to be achieved. For example, glucose dehydrogenase can be added to glucose oxidase, using NADH as a recycled substrate to generate additional O_2. Amplification factors ranging from 60 to over 200 times have been achieved for lactate biosensors using lactate oxidase with lactate dehydrogenase, based on recycling NADH to generate more O_2. Scott and Skillen (1992) coimmobilized lactate dehydrogenase and lactate oxidase on a trichlorotriazine-activated nylon membrane. A Pt anode, treated with 1% (w/v) Nafion diluted in dimethyl formamide in 5% alcohol, was used as an H_2O_2 transducer. The biosensor was found to be eight times more sensitive to NADH than previous tests with biosensors that had the enzymes on separate membranes. However, the biosensor life-time was not very good, with the sensitivity falling by about 50% in two weeks.

4.9.4 Inhibition of Enzyme Recycling

Seegopaul and Rechnitz (1984) developed and tested a biosensor for methotrexate, a therapeutic drug used in cancer treatment. The biosensor took advantage of the two-enzyme reaction

$$\text{dihydrofolate reductase}$$

$$\text{dihydrofolate} + \text{NADPH} \rightarrow \text{tetrahydrofolate} + \text{NADP}^+$$

$$\text{6-phosphogluconic dehydrogenase} \tag{102}$$

$$\text{NADP}^+ + \text{6-phosphogluconate} \rightarrow$$

$$\text{NADPH} + \text{ribulose-5-phosphate} + \text{CO}_2$$

since methotrexate inhibited the recycling of NADPH. The reaction was monitored with a CO_2 transducer, with a fall in CO_2 measured after inhibition. Optimum enzyme levels were chosen to insure that the overall rate of reaction was dependent on difolate reductase. The lower limit of detection was around 1.5 μg/L. In the range of clinical relevance up to 12 μg/L, the precision ranged between ± 1.9 to 5.2%. Above methotrexate levels around 15 μg/L, the biosensor became increasingly more nonlinear, eventually becoming relatively insensitive due to near maximal inhibition.

4.10 CARBON ELECTRODE ENZYME-BASED BIOSENSORS

4.10.1 Basic Theory

Carbon electrodes may be less sensitive to fouling effects, and may be more compatible with enzymes than noble metal electrodes, especially when operated in a pulse mode. Tarasevich and Khruschcheva (1989) propose the following reaction scheme

$$E + O_2 \rightarrow EO_2$$

$$EO_2 + e^- \rightarrow EO_2^- \tag{103}$$

for the reduction of O_2 on carbon catalyzed by an immobilized enzyme (E).

The rapid electron transfer for the second step probably stabilizes the EO_2 complex and facilitates its protonation in the following step

$$EO_2^- + H^+ \rightarrow EO_2H \tag{104}$$

The next two-electron step

$$EO_2H + 2e^- + H^+ \rightarrow EO^- + H_2O \tag{105}$$

may involve a slower tunnel mechanism for electron transfer between the active center of the enzyme through the carbon carrier to the acceptor sites on the O_2 molecule. The reaction proceeds with

$$EO^- + e^- + H^+ \rightarrow EOH^- \tag{106}$$

and

$$EOH^- + H^+ \rightarrow E + H_2O \tag{107}$$

for a net production of $2H_2O$ for each O_2 molecule reduced.

4.10.2 Applications

Tarasevich and Khruschcheva (1989) measured kinetic data for the reduction of O_2 on carbon blacks with immobilized laccase. The results were found to be consistent with the previous reaction scheme. Furthermore, a potential close to the equilibrium potential for O_2 could be used. Doblhoff-Dier and Rechnitz (1989) used three electrodes: glassy carbon working electrode, Pt counterelectrode, and a saturated calomel reference with a potentiostat for an amperometric method to determine superoxide dismutase activity (SOD). The principle of operation was based on the fact that SOD inhibits the reaction

$$xanthine\ oxidase$$

$$xanthine + O_2 + H_2O \rightarrow uric\ acid + H_2O_2 \tag{108}$$

This biosensor had a very simple design, with xanthine oxidase dissolved in 0.1 mM EDTA buffer at physiological pH in a 25 mL glass chamber. When the glassy carbon electrode potential was held at 0 V, Doblhoff-Dier and Rechnitz (1989) were able to detect a steady state current that they believed may have been directly due to superoxide radicals. Other chemical species could also be detected at positive (uric acid, H_2O_2) or negative (O_2) potentials as expected. Uric acid could be followed at $+0.45$ V. The bioassay procedure consisted of adding a known amount of xanthine (50 μM) to the chamber, to generate a steady state current with the potentiostat held at 0 V. Then a known amount of SOD was added, and the decrease in current due to inhibition was measured.

They found that the inhibition by SOD was independent of xanthine oxidase concentration $>4 \times 10^{-3}$ U/mL. A semi-logarithmic curve for SOD was found, with a lower limit of detection for SOD at 8×10^{-11} M when the pH $= 7$. They also found that the biosensor sensitivity depended on pH and type of buffer used. The lower limit of detection for SOD was 2×10^{-12} M at pH $= 9$. The same type of assay could be done with a known volume of tissue homogenate to determine SOD. This technique may be useful for measurements of this important free radical scavenger in tissues.

In addition to directly modified carbon electrodes, carbon pastes have been made by combining fine carbon particles with silicone oil, paraffin oil, Nujol, ceresin wax, and other materials. Enzymes may be immobilized on the carbon surface and electrically connected to noble metal or other types of electrodes. This approach was used in the rechargeable, implantable glucose biosensor designed by Xie and Wilkins (1991) which was described earlier in this section.

4.11 ORGANIC PHASE ENZYME BIOSENSORS

4.11.1 Basic Theory

It may be possible to lock some enzymes into a more active conformation by using organic liquids, such as benzene, chloroform, heptane, or hexane, instead of aqueous media. However, some trace amount of H_2O is required to insure that the enzyme retains its catalytic activity. Also, a nonaqueous support electrolyte or other method for transferring electrons in the organic phase is required, since most of the nonpolar organic liquids are generally nonconductive. This is a very recent concept for biosensors which may prove to be especially useful for analytes that are sparingly soluble in water, such as oils and lipids, and for medically relevant molecules such as cholesterol or bilirubin. Also, there is evidence that this technique can maintain some enzymes at a higher level of catalytic activity than is normally possible in H_2O. The organic phase may also significantly extend the lifetime of some enzymes compared to aqueous environments.

4.11.2 Applications

Saini et al. (1991) recently reviewed the relatively limited amount of research that has been conducted on biosensors using organic liquids. Hall et al. (1988) appear to be the first to successfully use this principle. They measured p-cresol using polyphenol oxidase coimmobilized with a support electrolyte, tetrabutylammoniumtoluene-4-sulfonate, dissolved in chloroform. The oxidase and support electrolyte were placed in a nylon mesh over a carbon electrode. The enzyme catalyzed the reaction of p-cresol to 4-methyl-1,2-benzoquinone, which could be reduced on the carbon electrode at -275 mV. The organic phase enzyme electrode was linear in the concentration range up to 0.1 M p-cresol, and was shown to be useful for measurements of p-cresol contamination in wastewater.

Hall and Turner (1990) developed an organic phase biosensor for cholesterol, using cholesterol oxidase immobilized on alumina powder in a 1:1 (v/v) mixture of chloroform and hexane. An O_2 electrode was used as the biosensor transducer. The optimum enzyme activity was obtained when there was 5% (v/v) H_2O present, which was thought to be associated primarily with the enzyme on the alumina powder. The biosensor was linear within the range of cholesterol concentration from 1 to 10 mM, with a lower detection limit around 0.4 mM. However, the biosensor was also sensitive to sterols. Schubert et al. (1991) developed an H_2O_2 biosensor by coimmobilizing horseradish peroxidase in chloroform along with potassium hexacyanoferrate(II), which can transfer electrons as it goes to the III form in the presence of H_2O_2 (see next section). The organic phase biosensor was linear up to 600 μM H_2O_2.

4.12 ALTERNATE ELECTRON DONORS

4.12.1 Basic Theory

While O_2 is the major biological source of free electrons for the maintenance of metabolic energy in animal cells, other redox agents can provide a source of electrons for the many different types of enzyme-catalyzed bioreactions discussed so far. A number of alternate electron donors have been investigated besides ferrocene derivatives, including various guinones, tetrathiafulvalene, tungsten complexes, ruthenium complexes, phenoxazines (such as alizarin green), phenothiazines (methylene green, methylene blue, azure A, B, or C) and conducting organic salts such as N-methylphenazinium (NMP$^+$) or 7,7,8,8-tetracyanoquinodimethane (TCNQ). Gorton et al. (1991) reviewed some of these applications for flow through systems.

An advantage for using an alternate electron transfer mediator is that the measurement can be made under hypoxic or anoxic conditions when O_2 is no longer available as the usual electron donor. Unfortunately, when O_2 is present, it may be able to successfully compete with the alternate electron donor and therefore act as an interfering chemical species. Another advantage for using an alternate electron donor in an amperometric biosensor, is that it may be possible to measure the current at a smaller overpotential than is normally required to operate either O_2 or H_2O_2 electrodes. This may also be helpful in minimizing interference from other substrates that might be reduced or oxidized at the higher overpotentials.

4.12.2 Applications

Cass et al. (1984) were the first to exploit the ferrocene and ferricinium redox couple

$$2Fe(CN)_6^{4-} \rightleftharpoons 2Fe(CN)_6^{3-} + 2e^- \tag{109}$$

to supply electrons in a glucose biosensor. The electron donor replaces O_2 in the reaction catalyzed by glucose oxidase [Equation (91)], as shown in Figure 4.4. Since then, many others have investigated the use of ferrocene derivatives for alternate electron donors in enzyme-based biosensors. For example, Kubiak and Wang (1989) tried to electrostatically immobilize potassium hexacyanoferrate ions by incorporating 5% poly-4-vinylpyridine (PVP) into a carbon paste. However, they reported that electrodes modified in this manner suffered from poor stability, which they attributed to the gradual loss of surface-bound ions.

Hale et al. (1991a) found that a dibenzylviologen derivative allowed the use of a more cathodic potential (-350 to -400 mV versus a saturated calomel electrode) for their glucose biosensor. This allowed the biosensor to be operated at a range where ascorbate and urate do not interfere with the measurement. Furthermore, this potential is close to the optimum for the glucose oxidase reaction around -450 mV. Generally, most investigators have found that higher current densities can be achieved with many of the electron donors. This allows lower detection limits with improved signal-to-noise ratios. However, the electron donor may be free to diffuse out of the membrane, eventually leading to reduced sensitivity of the biosensor. This problem was attributed to the one-third drop in sensitivity observed after one week by Kajiya et al. (1991) for their glucose biosensor, which used hydroquinonesulfonate ions electropolymerized with glucose oxidase in a polypyrrole film.

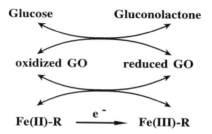

FIGURE 4.4. *Alternate pathway for electron transport in a glucose oxidase–catalyzed bioreaction with glucose through a ferrocene derivative redox mediator.*

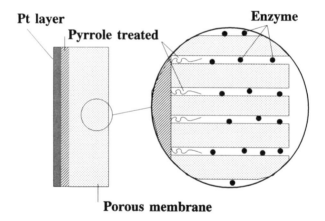

FIGURE 4.5. *Schematic drawing of an immobilized enzyme within the pores of a membrane with a layer of redox mediator (pyrrole). Electrons are detected by direct molecular connections from the redox mediator to a layer of vapor-deposited Pt. Koopal et al. (1991) constructed and tested a glucose biosensor using this design.*

4.12.3 Directly Wired Enzymes

Methods are currently being developed for cross-linking electron donors within conducting polymer membranes to directly "wire" the enzyme and electrochemical transducer together. For example, Gregg and Heller (1990) describe a one-step procedure for a glucose biosensor based on a poly-(vinylpyridine) complex of $Os(bpy)_2Cl$. This conducting polymer was quaternized using either a bromoacetic or a bromopropionic acid ester of *N*-hydroxysuccinimide to form electrostatic complexes with glucose oxidase. Presumably, amide bonds are formed on the lysine terminals of the enzyme. The polymer, ester, glucose oxidase and a cross-linking agent (trien) were mixed together and directly applied to Au, Pt, graphite, and glassy carbon electrodes. After drying under vacuum, the electrodes were uniformly covered with a thin conducting polymer film with excellent charge transfer properties. The competition between O_2 and the redox polymer was investigated. Although Gregg and Heller (1990) found that their conducting polymer glucose biosensors were still O_2 dependent, the dependence was estimated to be substantially less than would be found with conventional O_2 or H_2O_2 electrochemical transducers.

Koopal et al. (1991) coated one side of a filtration membrane with a conducting polypyrrole polymer, as shown in Figure 4.5. This side was then sputtered with Pt, forming a layer about 100 nm thick, to permit electrical contact when placed over a conventional Pt or carbon electrochemical transducer. Glucose oxidase was immobilized inside the 600 nm pores of the filtration membrane, as confirmed from microscopy using fluorescein-labeled enzyme, suggesting that direct connections were made between the polypyrrole and glucose oxidase. Good stability after two weeks was observed with this hybrid type of membrane biosensor. Hale et al. (1991b) tested seven different types of methyl hydrosiloxane and dimethylsiloxane copolymers for their effectiveness in covalently attaching ferrocene and glucose oxidase in graphite powder pastes. The highest current densities were found with type II and III copolymers. However, the biosensors were still sensitive to O_2. About 20% loss in sensitivity was found after 220 days when stored dry at $4°C$, with significantly greater losses when stored wet.

4.13 REFERENCES

Arnold, M. A. and M. E. Meyerhoff. 1988. "Recent Advances in the Development and Analytical Applications of Biosensing Probes," *C.R.C. Crit. Rev. Anal. Chem.*, 20:149–196.

Bardeletti, G., F. Séchaud and P. R. Coulet. 1991. "Amperometric Enzyme Electrodes for Substrate and Enzyme Activity Determinations," in *Biosensor Principles and Applications*, L. J. Blum and P. R. Coulet, eds., New York, NY: M. Dekker, Inc., pp. 7–45.

Buerk, D. G. 1990. "Oxygen Control of Oxidative Metabolism" (letter to editor), *J. Appl. Physiol.*, 69:2318–2319.

Buerk, D. G., P. K. Nair and W. J. Whalen. 1989a. "Two-Cytochrome Model for Carotid Body $P_{t_i}O_2$ and Chemosensitivity Changes after Hemorrhage," *J. Appl. Physiol.*, 67:60–66.

Buerk, D. G., P. K. Nair and W. J. Whalen. 1989b. "Evidence for Second Metabolic Pathway for O_2 from $P_{t_i}O_2$ Measurements in Denervated Cat Carotid Body," *J. Appl. Physiol.*, 67:1578–1584.

Cass, A. E. G., G. Davis, G. D. Francis and H. A. O. Hill. 1984. "Ferrocene-Mediated Enzyme Electrode for Amperometric Determination of Glucose," *Anal. Chem.*, 56:667–671.

Clark, L. C., Jr. 1973. "A Polarographic Enzyme Electrode for the Measurement of Oxidase Substrates," in *Oxygen Supply—Theoretical and Practical Aspects of Oxygen Supply and Microcirculation of Tissue*, M. Kessler, D. F. Bruley, L. C. Clark, Jr., D. W. Lübbers, I. A. Silver and J. Strauss, eds., W. Germany: Urban and Schwarzenberg, pp. 120–128.

Clark, L. C., Jr. and C. Lyons. 1962. "Electrode Systems for Continuous Monitoring in Cardiovascular Surgery," *Ann. N. Y. Acad. Sci.*, 102:29.

Coulet, P. R., G. Bardeletti and F. Séchaud. 1991. "Amperometric Enzyme Membrane Electrodes," in *Bioinstrumentation and Biosensors*, D. L. Wise, ed., New York, NY: M. Dekker, Inc., pp. 753–793.

Doblhoff-Dier, O. and G. A. Rechnitz. 1989. "Amperometric Method for the Determination of Superoxide Dismutase Activity at Physiological pH," *Anal. Chim. Acta.*, 222: 247–252.

Garber, C. C., J. O. Westgard, L. Milz and F. C. Larson. 1982. "DuPont ACA III Performance as Tested According to NCCLS Guidelines," *Clin. Chem.*, 25:1730–1738.

Gorton, L., E. Csöregi, E. Domínguez, J. Emnéus, G. Jönsson-Pettersson, G. Marko-Varga and B. Persson. 1991. "Selective Detection in Flow Analysis Based on the Combination of Immobilized Enzymes and Chemically Modified Electrodes," *Anal. Chim. Acta*, 250:203–248.

Gough, D. A., J. Y. Lucisano and P. H. S. Tse. 1985. "Two-Dimensional Enzyme Electrode Sensor for Glucose," *Anal. Chem.*, 57:2351–2357.

Gregg, B. A. and A. Heller. 1990. "Cross-Linked Redox Gels Containing Glucose Oxidase for Amperometric Biosensor Applications," *Anal. Chem.*, 62:258–263.

Guilbault, G. G. 1973. "Enzyme Electrodes for Biomedical Analysis," *Vol. II, Digest, 10th Conf. Med. and Biol. Eng., Dresden, W. Germany*, p. 54.

Guilbault, G. G. and J. G. Montalvo. 1969. "A Urea-Specific Enzyme Electrode," *J. Am. Chem. Soc.*, 91:2164.

Guilbault, G. G. and F. R. Shu. 1972. "Enzyme Electrodes Based on the Use of a Carbon Dioxide Sensor: Urea and L-Tyrosine Electrodes," *Anal. Chem.*, 44:2161.

Guilbault, G. G., B. Danielsson, C. F. Mandenius and K. Mosbach. 1983. "A Comparison of Enzyme Electrode and Thermistor Probes for Assay of Alcohols Using Alcohol Oxidase," *Anal. Chem.*, 55:1582–1585.

Guilbault, G. G., A. A. Suleiman, O. Fatibello-Filho and M. A. NabiRahni. 1991. "Immobilized Bioelectrochemical Sensors," in *Bioinstrumentation and Biosensors*, D. L. Wise, ed., New York, NY: M. Dekker, Inc., pp. 659–692.

Hale, P. D., L. I. Boguslavsky, T. Inagaki, H. I. Karan, H. S. Lee, T. A. Skotheim and Y.

Okamoto. 1991b. "Amperometric Glucose Biosensors Based on Redox Polymer-Mediated Electron Transfer," *Anal. Chem.*, 63:667–682.

Hale, P. D., L. I. Boguslavsky, H. I. Karan, H. L. Lan, H. S. Lee, Y. Okamoto and T. A. Skotheim. 1991a. "Investigation of Viologen Derivatives as Electron-Transfer Mediators in Amperometric Glucose Sensors," *Anal. Chim. Acta*, 248:155–161.

Hall, G. F. 1988. "The Determination of *p*-Cresol in Chloroform with an Enzyme Electrode Used in the Organic Phase," *Anal. Chim. Acta*, 213:113–119.

Hall, G. F. and A. P. F. Turner. 1990. In *Biosensors '90. First World Conference on Biosensors, Elsevier Seminars, Oxford, Great Britain*, p. 331.

Janata, J. and A. Bezegh. 1988. "Chemical Sensors," *Anal. Chem.*, 60:62R–74R.

Kajiya, Y., H. Sugai, C. Iwakura and H. Yoneyama. 1991. "Glucose Sensitivity of Polypyrrole Films Containing Immobilized Glucose Oxidase and Hydroquinonesulfonate Ions," *Anal. Chem.*, 63:49–54.

Kauffman, J-M. and G. G. Guilbault. 1991. "Potentiometric Enzyme Electrodes," in *Biosensor Principles and Applications*, L. J. Blum and P. R. Coulct, eds., New York, NY: M. Dekker, Inc., pp. 63–82.

Koopal, C. J. G., B. deRuiter and R. J. M. Nolte. 1991. "Amperometric Biosensor Based on Direct Communication between Glucose Oxidase and A Conducting Polymer inside the Pores of a Filtration Membrane," *J. Chem. Soc. Chem. Commun.*, 23:1691–1692.

Kumaran, S., H. Meier, A. M. Danna and C. Tran-Minh. 1991. "Immobilization of Thin Enzyme Membranes to Construct Glass Enzyme Electrodes," *Anal. Chem.*, 63:1914–1918.

Lubrano, G. J., M. H. Faridnia, G. Palleschi and G. G. Guilbault. 1991. "Amperometric Alcohol Electrode with Extended Linearity and Reduced Interferences," *Anal. Biochem.*, 198:97–103.

Macholán, L. 1991. "Biocatalytic Membrane Electrodes," in *Bioinstrumentation and Biosensors*, D. L. Wise, ed., New York, NY: M. Dekker, Inc., pp. 329–378.

McCall, A. L. and C. J. Mullin. 1986. "Home Monitoring of Diabetes Mellitus—A Quiet Revolution," *Clin. Lab. Med.*, 6:215–239.

Nilsson, H., A. Akerlund and K. Mosbach. 1973. "Determination of Glucose, Urea and Penicillin Using Enzyme-pH Electrodes," *Biochem. Biophys. Acta*, 320:529.

Pickup, J. C. 1989. "Biosensors for Diabetes Mellitus," in *Applied Biosensors*, D. L. Wise, ed., Boston, MA: Butterworths, pp. 227–247.

Saini, S., G. F. Hall, M. E. A. Downs and A. P. F. Turner. 1991. "Organic Phase Enzyme Electrodes," *Anal. Chim. Acta*, 249:1–15.

Scott, D. A. and A. W. Skillen. 1992. "Amperometric Enzyme Electrode for NADH Detection Employing Co-Immobilized Lactate Dehydrogenase and Lactate Oxidase," *Anal. Chim. Acta*, 256:47–52.

Schubert, F., U. Wollenberger, F. W. Scheller and H.-G. Müller. 1991. "Artificially Coupled Reactions with Immobilized Enzymes: Biological Analogs and Technical Consequences," in *Bioinstrumentation and Biosensors*, D. L. Wise, ed., New York, NY: M. Dekker, Inc., pp. 19–37.

Seegopaul, P. and G. A. Rechnitz. 1984. "Enzyme-Amplified Determination of Methotrexate with a pCO₂ Membrane Electrode," *Anal. Chem.*, 56:852–854.

Shichiri, M., N. Asakawa, Y. Yamasaki, R. Kanamori and H. Abe. 1986. "Telemetry Glucose Monitoring Device with Needle-Type Glucose Sensor: A Useful Tool for Blood Glucose Monitoring in Diabetic Individuals," *Diabetes Care*, 9:298–301.

Sode, K., E. Tamiya, I. Karube and Y. Kameda. 1989. "Sensor for Free Fatty Acids Based on Acyl Coenzyme-A Synthetase and Acyl Coenzyme-A Oxidase," *Anal. Chem. Acta*, 220:251–255.

Tarasevich, M. R. and E. I. Khruschcheva. 1989. "Electrocatalytic Properties of Carbon Materials," in *Modern Aspects of Electrochemistry—No. 19*, B. E. Conway, J. O.'M. Bockris and R. E. White, eds., New York, NY: Plenum Press, pp. 295–358.

Updike, S. J. and G. P. Hicks. 1967. "The Enzyme Electrode, A Miniature Chemical Transducer Using Immobilized Enzyme Activity," *Nature (Lond.)*, 214:986–988.

Updike, S. J., M. C. Schults, C. C. Capelli, D. von Heimburg, R. K. Rhodes, N. Joseph-Tipton, B. Anderson and D. D. Koch. 1988. "Laboratory Evaluation of New Reusable Blood Glucose Sensor," *Diabetes Care*, 11:801–807.

White, R. I., L. R. Waite, S. P. Lim and C. Spieker. 1991. "A Catheter-Based Enzyme-Coupled Electrode for Measurement of Lactate," *Biomed. Instrum. Technol.* (Nov./Dec.):461–464.

Watanabe, E. and M. Tanaka. 1991. "Determination of Fish Freshness with a Biosensor System," in *Bioinstrumentation and Biosensors*, D. L. Wise, ed., New York, NY: M. Dekker, Inc., pp. 39–73.

Wilkins, E. S. 1989. "Toward Implantable Glucose Sensors: A Review," *J. Biomed. Eng.*, 11:354–361.

Vanderkooi, J., M. Erecińska and I. A. Silver. 1991. "Oxygen in Mammalian Tissue: Methods of Measurement and Affinities of Various Reactions," *Am. J. Physiol.*, 260; *Cell Physiol.*, 29:C1131–C1150.

Xie, S.-L. and E. Wilkins. 1991. "Performances of Potentially Implantable Rechargeable Glucose Sensors *in vitro* at Body Temperature," *Biomed. Instrum. Technol.* (Sept./Oct.):393–399.

CHAPTER 5

Fabrication and Miniaturization Techniques

There can be both advantages and disadvantages in miniaturizing transducers that are commonly used for biosensors. For discrete sampling instruments, small sample volumes are often desirable. Detailed spatial resolution may be required for some applications. If the biosensor is intended for direct measurements in living tissues, it must be small enough to minimize damage to the cells or to the microcirculation in the tissue. If placed directly into the bloodstream, it must not impede blood flow. Smaller devices may be less durable and easier to break than larger ones. Finally, miniaturized transducers often have much more rapid response times than are possible with larger devices. However, the signals may also be smaller and more difficult to detect from miniaturized devices. A great amount of research effort has been spent in developing reliable fabrication techniques for miniaturizing electrochemical and optical transducers for conventional types of measurements as well as for biosensors.

5.1 MICROELECTRODES

5.1.1 Glass Micropipettes

There are a wide variety of microelectrodes made from pulled glass micropipettes, which can be used to make highly detailed spatial measurements. Various modifications to create specific types of microelectrodes are described in the following subsections. A brief history of the scientific applications for early glass micropipette techniques is summarized in a book by Brown and Flaming (1986). Most of these applications were for the measurement of intracellular membrane potentials and action potentials through simple glass microelectrodes filled with physiological salt solutions. Ling and Gerard (1949) were the first to use these types of microelectrodes for cell membrane potential measurements. Muscle and nerve cell electrophysiology owes its current understanding to this early research. Brown and Flaming (1986) also describe fabrication techniques and mechanical devices developed over the years to pull out glass micropipette tips with submicron dimensions.

5.1.2 Beveling

Glass micropipettes are usually beveled for two reasons. First, the tip is sharper and can better penetrate into tissue or cells. Second, the increased area of opening lowers the electrical resistance of the tip, or reduces the hydraulic resistance for pipettes used to microinject fluids. Mechanical grinding techniques are most frequently used. Barrett and Whitlock (1973) used a quartz rod painted with diamond dust particles <0.25 μm. Brown and Flaming (1974) used an optically flat glass plate coated with a polyurethane film that was dusted with alumina powder (diameters around 0.05 μm) when the film was still tacky. Commercial devices are now available which use a wobble-free, rotating surface coated with either diamond or alumina particles. The grinding surface can be used either wet or dry. Often the grinding surface is covered with a layer of saline or other electrically conductive ionic solution, which is grounded via an Ag/AgCl reference electrode. The tip size of saline-filled microelectrodes for cell membrane potential or neurophysiological measurements can be carefully controlled by monitoring their electrical resistance as the tips are ground. When micropipette tip diameters are around 0.1 μm, the electrical resistance is approximately 150 MΩ, falling to around 20 MΩ when the tip size increases to 0.5 μm (Brown and Flaming, 1974).

Different grinding techniques other than rotating solid surfaces have also been developed. Lederer et al. (1979) used a thick sediment of alumina powder that settled to the bottom of a rotating petri dish as a grinding surface. The sediment was covered with a KCl solution, so the electrical resistance of the microelectrode could be measured. Ogden et al. (1978) used a suspension of alumina powder in saline. A pressurized fluid reservoir forced the suspension through a hypodermic needle. Micropipettes were placed into the center of the flowing stream to abrade the tip. By grounding the fluid in the reservoir, the electrical resistance of the micropipette could be monitored.

5.1.3 Tip Measurements

Since the limit of resolution by light microscopy is around 0.4 μm due to light diffraction, tip dimensions of ultrafine microelectrodes cannot be accurately measured through the light microscope. A number of investigators have used scanning electron micrography to measure tip dimensions. This technique requires coating the microelectrode with gold or gold-palladium by RF vacuum sputtering. After coating with metal, some types of micro-electrodes using glass micropipettes may no longer be usable for electro-chemical measurements. Also, there is still some uncertainty in the mea-surement, since the thickness of the vapor-deposited metal coating must be subtracted to determine the true tip and glass wall dimensions. The actual coating thickness may not be precisely known or may not be uniform. Fry (1975) was able to examine uncoated glass micropipettes using the transmis-sion mode for scanning. In this case, the same microelectrode could be reused after making the measurements of wall thickness and tip dimen-sions.

Tip diameters of empty glass micropipettes have been measured by deter-mining the pressure required to form gas bubbles through the tip when it is submerged in water. The bubble count method, involving the number of bubbles within a given time produced by forcing air through a syringe, has been a technique for checking the consistency of micropipette dimensions after pulling (Mittman et al., 1987). Recently, Lissilour and Godinot (1990) measured the threshold pressure for compressed nitrogen gas to form bub-bles through micropipettes submerged in methanol. Methanol was used since the gas/liquid surface tension (22.2×10^{-3} Newton/meter) is much lower than for air and water (72×10^{-3} Newton/meter). Tip sizes between 0.2 to 5.0 μm were tested. Both the inner and outer diameters of the tip opening were determined and confirmed later by scanning electron micros-copy. They found a least squares fit to a double log plot of the measured pressure and tip dimensions, with the following result

$$D = \frac{3.172 \times \text{surface tension}}{P^{1.01}} \tag{110}$$

where D is the inner tip diameter and the pressure P is in Pascals (Newton/ m^2). The relationship is essentially the LaPlace equation for surface ten-sion, except that the exponent 1.01 was found experimentally rather than 1 expected from theory. Hence, a pressure of 310 kPa (a little over three at-mospheres) is required to pass bubbles into methanol through a tip with an inner diameter of 0.2 μm. The pressure to pass bubbles into water through the same size tip would be 995 kPa (nearly 10 atmospheres).

5.1.4 Single-Barrel pH Microelectrodes

Glass pH electrodes have been miniaturized using several different microelectrode designs, as illustrated in Figure 5.1. The simplest design

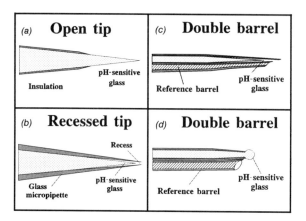

FIGURE 5.1. *Schematic drawings for several different glass-sensitive pH microelectrodes developed by (a) Hinke (1967), (b) Thomas (1974), (c) DeHemptinne (1980) and (d) Javaheri et al. (1985).*

was an open tip microelectrode, made by pulling out pH-sensitive glass. In the early 1950s, Caldwell (1956) fabricated a 50–80 μm diameter glass electrode and attempted to measure intracellular pH in large crab muscle fibers and giant squid axons. However, the pH-sensitive part of the electrode was at least 500 mm long. Measurements were made by inserting the electrode horizontally into the fibers, and probably caused significant tissue damage. A smaller, 20 μm diameter pH electrode was constructed by Hinke (1967). He improved the open-tip design by insulating the glass shaft as much as possible, as shown schematically in Figure 5.1(a). His new design still had an open tip with a relatively long length of pH-sensitive glass, around 150 μm. With such a long length, it was not possible to make true intracellular pH measurements except in exceptionally large cells.

Thomas (1974) made a recessed-tip pH microelectrode, shown schematically in Figure 5.1(b), which offered a significant improvement over previous open-tip types. A pH glass microelectrode was pulled out, then inserted into a second glass micropipette which insulated the inner glass from H^+ ions. By applying mechanical pressure and local heating with a microforge, the two micropipettes could be fused together. The pH-sensitive glass was thus protected inside a recess, with the tip of the external glass micropipette made < 1 μm. These small dimensions permitted the spatial resolution that is necessary for intracellular pH measurements. However, one drawback of this design was a longer time response compared to open tips due to the increased diffusion distance in the recess from the tip to the pH transducer. Also, the measured EMF must be corrected for the cell membrane potential if an intracellular measurement is made with the reference electrode external to the cell.

5.1.5 Double-Barrel pH Microelectrodes

DeHemptinne (1980) modified the glass pH electrode by using a double-barrel design, shown schematically in Figure 5.1(c). The design combines the recessed Thomas-type pH glass tip with a second barrel, which is used as the reference electrode. This microelectrode could be placed intracellularly if the dimensions were sufficiently small. A more open tip type of double-barrel pH sensor is described by Javaheri et al. (1985), which is shown schematically in Figure 5.1(d). The construction methods are rather complex, although they claim these microelectrodes are relatively easy to make.

First, a double-barrel micropipette was pulled from borosilicate glass. One barrel is used as the reference and the other for an insulator. A second micropipette was then pulled from pH-sensitive glass (Corning 0150), and the tip was melted with a microforge to form a blunter end. The pH glass micropipette was then inserted inside one of the borosilicate glass barrels and advanced upwards towards the tip. The two tips were then fused together by local heating with the microforge while applying pressure inside the pH glass with a compressed gas source. This expanded the pH glass to a slightly larger tip size as it was heated, filling the space inside the outer pipette. After the two glass pipettes were fused together, the pH glass pipette was mechanically advanced, until the fused tip fractured and fell off. The glass pH micropipette was then advanced further until the broken tip protruded out of the borosilicate glass. The tip was again melted, closing the end of the pH-sensitive glass, and fusing the pH and borosilicate glass together. By again applying pressure from the compressed gas source during local heating, a small bulb of the pH-sensitive glass was made, which protrudes from the insulating barrel, as shown in Figure 5.1(d).

The pH-sensitive barrel was filled with 0.1 M NaCl buffered to pH 6 with 0.1 M citrate buffer, taking care to eliminate any bubbles. The second reference barrel was filled with an ionic solution similar to the extracellular fluid of the tissue under study, to reduce liquid junction potentials. Typical tip dimensions were reported to be between 10 to 35 μm for the pH bulb, and about one-third smaller for the reference barrel. Extracellular pH measurements in brain tissue were made with this type of sensor.

5.1.6 Ion-Sensitive Microelectrodes

Fabrication details for ion-sensitive microelectrodes using liquid neutral carrier ionophores in glass micropipettes are described in the book by Ammann (1986). Earlier types of ion-sensitive microelectrodes used ion exchange resins, which tended to have very high electrical resistances compared to more recent neutral carrier ionophore types. Both single-barrel and double-barrel designs have been used by various investigators.

The micropipettes are usually beveled first. Then the glass tip must be treated to reduce its normally hydrophilic properties, which are caused by a relatively high density of hydroxyl groups on the glass surface. This can be accomplished by silanization, usually with a reactive silicon compound (chlorosilanes, aminosilanes, or siloxanes) dissolved in an organic liquid, such as carbon tetrachloride. Silicon oils have also been used with some success. Various silanization techniques have been investigated, including simple dipping in liquid silanes, or heating to produce vapors that reach inside the tip. The silanization step is thought to produce covalent bonding to the glass surface, which creates a more stable interface inside the tip for retaining the liquid containing the neutral carrier ionophore.

The neutral carrier ionophore can be introduced into the tip either by suction or from the back using high pressure to push it forward. The microelectrode is then back-filled with a solution that contains the specific ion of interest. The magnitude of the Nernst potential that results will depend on the difference between the back-filled concentration and the external ion concentration near the tip [Equation (70)] and may also be sensitive to other interfering ions. The microelectrode must be stored in the same solution, and has a limited lifetime due to degradation of the ionophore and leakage from the tip. Interference from other ions is possible, and measurements must be corrected for junction potentials if they are present. When intracellular measurements are made, the membrane potential of the cell must be subtracted from the total EMF. As discussed previously in Chapter 3, there are commercial neutral carrier ionophores available for over thirty anions and cations.

A new type of microhole design for an ionic transducer was described by Abatti and Moriizumi (1992). The construction method combines conventional glass micropipettes with a photolithographic method. A microhole was created in a 1,500 Å thick film of silicon nitride (Si_3N_4) by electron beam and reactive ion etching. A borosilicate glass tube was preheated, then bonded to the film, using a ring etched into the film as a guide to centering the microhole. A two-step process was used, applying heat before and after contact with the film to insure good bonding. The new geometrical design was tested as a K^+ ion transducer using a neutral carrier ionophore, with the body filled with a KCl solution. The body of the microelectrode had much thicker glass walls and was physically much larger than conventional pulled micropipettes, so the new design is not suitable for making intracellular measurements.

5.1.7 pH and Ion Measurement

All of the glass micropipette pH- and ion-sensitive microelectrodes described previously tend to have very high electrical resistances, requiring high input impedances for the amplifiers that measure their EMF. Careful electromagnetic shielding is needed to improve the signal-to-noise ratio. A major disadvantage of glass pH electrodes is the rather long time response compared to other pH sensors. The time response can be shortened by grinding the glass to make it thinner at the sensor tip, but there must be a tradeoff with the reduced mechanical strength and greater fragility of the glass tip. Of course, glass micropipettes are very fragile, and measurements cannot be made for physiological conditions where there is excessive movement. For the liquid neutral carrier type of microelectrodes, the equivalent pore radius and pore length for ionic movements determine the time response. Microcracks in the very thin glass walls near the tip can have an effect on the resistance and capacitance. The thick wall microhole ion transducer designed by Abatti and Moriizumi (1992) described previously was found to have a lower resistance and junction potential, and a more stable capacitance than conventional pulled glass micropipette types of ion-sensitive microelectrodes.

5.1.8 Metal Microelectrodes

Etched metal wire microelectrodes, such as the one shown schematically in Figure 5.2(a), are much more durable than glass micropipettes. Wolbarsht et al. (1960) appear to be the first to use an electrochemical etching technique to produce metal microelectrodes with very fine points. Platinum-iridium (70:30) wire was etched by an AC source in a solution of 50% sodium cyanide with 30% sodium hydroxide added to prevent formation of cyanide gas. The bath was agitated during the initial shaping of the wire, which was carried out at 6 to 10 V relative to a carbon rod reference electrode. For the final electropolishing step, a much smaller voltage of 0.8 V was used, without agitating the bath. The taper was controlled by the amount of wire left submerged in the bath. After etching, the final tip size was $< 1 \ \mu$m. Others have used a mechanical dipping process in combination with electrolysis to produce more finely tapered metal microelectrodes. Although the microelectrodes fabricated by Wolbarsht et al. (1960) were intended for use in electrophysiological measurements, identical etching techniques have been used to fabricate needle-type microelectrodes to make electrochemical measurements of O_2, H_2 gas, H_2O_2, or other chemical species.

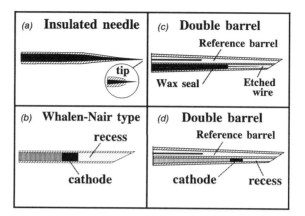

FIGURE 5.2. *Schematic drawings for O_2 microelectrodes designed by (a) Wolbarsht et al. (1960), (b) Whalen et al. (1967), (c) Tsacopoulos and Lehmenkühler (1977), and (d) Whalen et al. (1973).*

5.1.9 Insulation

After cleaning in distilled water and thorough drying, the etched metal microelectrodes were coated except at the very tip as shown in Figure 5.2(a) with glass heated to the melting point in a microforge. The tip was pushed into the molten drop of glass, then the shaft was advanced through it. Wolbarsht et al. (1960) used a low melting point solder glass (Corning 7570) which could be worked at 560°C. A higher melting point (990°C) potash lead glass (Corning 0041) was also tried, but less uniform coatings were obtained. To keep the glass workable, it was necessary to increase the electrical heating of the glass drop as the larger shank of the electrode moved upwards, due to increased thermal losses. After coating, it was sometimes necessary to fracture a thin glass layer at the tip by briefly passing a high current through it. Other plastic or polymer electrical insulators can be coated on the microelectrode. Parylene has been found to be a good insulating material, and is commonly used for neural recording or stimulating microelectrodes. Besides Pt, other metal wires can be etched and insulated. For example, a glass-insulated etched antimony wire was used by Vieira and Malnic (1968) to make the first true pH microelectrode for studies of H^+ ion secretion in the kidney.

5.1.10 Nanodes

Recently, Penner et al. (1990) modified the fabrication technique for bare-tip glass-coated Pt microelectrodes to produce spatial resolution at the nanometer scale. The extremely small dimensions of these ultramicroelectrodes, which they called nanodes, were assessed by scanning electron microscopy at 50,000 times magnification. The basic fabrication technique of the wire by electrochemical etching and glass coating was essentially the same as used by Wolbarsht et al. (1960). The glass coating was made by heating a glass bead up to between 1,250 and 1,370°C on a microforge, then moving the bare metal etched wire at a constant translation velocity through the molten glass. After coating, some of the microelectrodes had bare tips with <0.5 μm diameters, which were similar to the earlier bare-tip needle types. However, some tips appeared to be completely covered with glass. Even so, a pathway must have been available for molecular movement, probably through a very small channel in the glass. About 10% of these nanodes exhibited sensitivity to apparent electrochemical radii in the range from 10 to 100 Å. Although the currents measured with such tiny microelectrodes were extremely small, the effective current densities were quite large. Penner et al. (1990) estimated effective current densities around 70 A/cm^2. Much faster rates of electron transfer could be measured with these tiny nanodes compared to microelectrodes with larger tips. In fact, the smallest nanode they tested, which had an apparent chemical radius of 10 Å, was estimated to be capable of measuring kinetic rate constants within a factor of six of the theoretical upper limit for a single Pt atom, which has a radius of 1.53 Å.

5.1.11 Recessed Metal Alloy Microelectrodes

The recessed cathode PO$_2$ microelectrode fabricated by Whalen et al. (1967) combines glass micropipette and metal electrode designs, and can produce microelectrodes with longer tapers and greater mechanical flexibility than glass-coated etched metal wires. A schematic drawing for the recessed microelectrode design is shown in Figure 5.2(b). After pulling out a conventional glass micropipette and beveling the tip, it is filled with a low melting point metal alloy, such as Wood's metal (tin, antimony, and bismuth). Some of the metal alloy is removed from the tip by electrochemical etching in cyanide to form a recess approximately 20 to 50 μm deep. The alloy can be electroplated with noble metals such as gold or platinum. The tip is submerged into the plating solution, allowing sufficient time to completely fill the recess. A gold cathode 10 to 20 μm thick is plated onto the metal at 1 V, leaving a recess length at least 10 times the tip diameter. The tip is then soaked in distilled water to remove all plating solution. A hydrophobic membrane can be introduced into the recess by soaking in a dilute aqueous solution of Rhoplex polymer (Rohm and Haas), then drying. Dry microelectrodes can be stored indefinitely, but the membrane must be rehydrated in saline or distilled water before use. Polarographic currents for recessed PO_2 microelectrodes typically range from 10^{-11} to 10^{-10} amp in room-air equilibrated saline. Response times for 90% completion of a step change in PO_2 are <100 msec. Tip dimensions are typically <2 μm.

Nair et al. (1985) plated antimony for a metal oxide pH sensor using the recessed microelectrode design. Earlier, Satake et al. (1980) had examined the O_2 sensitivity [Equation (62)] of 2 to 5 μm diameter, bare-tipped antimony microelectrodes, finding a slope ($dE/d \log_{10} PO_2$) of 11.7 mV in the PO_2 range from 6 to 101 kPa (45 to 760 Torr). Kiani and Schubert (1988) tested bare and recessed antimony oxide pH microelectrodes and found that recessing reduced the degree of O_2 interference. The recess probably acts as a relative diffusion barrier, restricting the amount of O_2 that can reach the surface. The antimony oxide pH microelectrode was used by Nair et al. (1986) to make measurements of gerbil brain pH changes during cerebral ischemia. The author has been using a similar pH microelectrode for measurements in the cat eye. Palladium is plated into the recess rather than antimony, to further minimize the possibility for O_2 interference.

5.1.12 Double-Barrel Microelectrodes

A double-barrel O_2 microelectrode was designed by Tsacopoulos and Lehmenkühler (1977) with an etched Pt wire sealed with wax in one barrel, as shown schematically in Figure 5.2(c). The second barrel was filled with physiological saline. Examples for simultaneous measurements of PO_2 and bioelectrical activity in rat brain and in the honeybee retina using this microelectrode design were also described. The Whalen-Nair metal alloy filled, recessed cathode PO_2 microelectrode has also been fabricated in a double-barrel configuration, shown schematically in Figure 5.2(d). Whalen et al. (1976) used a spring-mounted, "floating" double-barrel microelectrode to measure simultaneous cardiac action potentials and tissue PO_2 in the beating cat heart.

Linsenmeier and Yancey (1987) used a double-barrel microelectrode for PO_2 and electrophysiological potential measurements in the cat eye. They described a technique for producing the recess that may be easier than removing alloy by electrochemical etching. One barrel was back-filled by heating a thin wire of metal alloy that has a low melting temperature. The wire was made by sucking molten metal into Teflon tubing with a slightly smaller diameter than the glass tube. After cooling, the Teflon was stripped off. The wire was pushed into the pipette as it melted, removing heat just before complete filling, leaving a recess >50 μm from the tip. The cathode was plated as described previously. Combined tip diameters can be made <5 μm for double-barrel microelectrodes using either method of construction. Double-barrel microelectrodes must be stored wet, preferably in the same solution that the second barrel is filled with.

The author is presently fabricating and evaluating double-barrel recessed microelectrodes where both barrels are filled with metal alloy. Combined PO_2 and pH microelectrodes are made by plating gold in one barrel and palladium in the other. Another design variation is also being developed by the author, where one barrel is metal filled and the second barrel is filled with a neutral carrier ionophore for ion measurements.

5.1.13 Carbon Fiber Microelectrodes

Recently, fine carbon fibers (7 to 12 μm diameter) have been used to construct microelectrodes to measure neurotransmitters and their metabolites *in vivo*. The carbon fiber is placed into a glass micropipette, fixing the fiber in the tip by sealing the lower shank with epoxy or another suitable adhesive. A bare length of fiber is left exposed from the tip. Electrical contact with the carbon fiber is made by back-filling the upper part of the electrode body with mercury, carbon paste, or an electrolyte solution. Conductive silver paint is another common technique for making electrical connection to the carbon fiber. An Ag/AgCl or other metal wire is placed into the conductive medium for connection to the amplifying electronics. A large Ag/AgCl wire in an agar bridge may be used as the reference electrode, or a second auxiliary electrode with an electrolyte-filled microelectrode connected by an Ag/AgCl wire can be used.

Although an untreated carbon surface can be used to detect catecholamine neurotransmitters (dopamine, norepinephrine, epinephrine) by high-speed cyclic voltammetric methods, the high reactivity of the oxidized chemical species tends to form electroinactive films on the surface which progressively diminish the electrode sensitivity. Furthermore, other oxidized chemical species can interfere with the measurement. Ascorbic acid, which plays an important antioxidant protective role by removing free radical products in brain tissue, and uric acid are the major interfering chemical species when measurements *in vivo* are made.

5.1.14 Chemically Modified Carbon Surfaces

Coury et al. (1989) reviewed some of the methods that have been used to chemically modify carbon fiber microelectrode surfaces in order to minimize the problems discussed previously. Electrochemical methods have been used to deliberately change the composition of the carbon oxides on the electrode surface. Electrodes that have been pretreated by alternating between periodic and steady voltage waveforms appear to have enhanced sensitivity to dopamine. Also, the oxidation potential for ascorbic acid is shifted to a more negative potential. This latter effect allows simultaneous measurement of ascorbic acid and catecholamines, if a suitable voltage waveform is applied to resolve the different oxidation reactions. Linear sweep voltammograms have been experimentally recorded from dopamine-rich areas of mammalian brain. Typically, three separate peaks are seen which are associated with ascorbic acid, uric acid, and homovanillic acid, a metabolite of dopamine. Another approach is to prevent ascorbic acid and uric acid from reaching the carbon surface. An anion-repelling hydrophobic agent such as stearic acid has been used for this purpose.

Rice and Nicholson (1989) used Nafion, a perfluorosulfonated polymer (DuPont) to coat carbon fiber microelectrodes. Nafion creates an ionomer membrane that has a large permeability difference between oppositely charged ionic species. Selectivity also appears to be improved by adding catecholamines to the liquid Nafion polymer prior to coating. Rice and Nicholson (1989) reported that the selectivity of dopamine relative to ascorbic acid was increased from about 30:1 for untreated carbon fiber microelectrodes to 2,200:1 after a single dip-coating of Nafion. They also applied a steady 0.5 V potential for 30 seconds while the tip was immersed in a drop of liquid Nafion to electrochemically pretreat the carbon surface. Although dopamine selectivity was greatly enhanced by these techniques, they also reported that this effect was not permanent. The selectivity fell markedly to about 160:1 for electrodes that were retested after they had been previously calibrated, rinsed with distilled water, and dried. Other researchers have reported that both electrochemically pretreated and Nafion-coated electrodes have greatly reduced sensitivities after they are used for brain studies.

5.1.15 Electrical and Heat Modified Carbon Surfaces

Another common technique for improving carbon fiber microelectrode performance is to pass current through the tip. Swain and Kuwana (1992) recently described differences in electrochemical behavior of carbon fiber after electrical and vacuum heat treatment. A bundle of about 3,000 individual fibers was first heat treated, then anodized by passing a 3.3 mA current through the bundle in acidic phosphate buffer (pH 2.2). This step was found to create fiber fractures and increased surface roughness, based on scanning electron microscopy. This also greatly increased the fiber capacitance by a factor of 1,000 or more, based on differential pulse voltammetric measurements in phosphate buffers made before and after treatment. Cyclic scan voltammetric measurements of dopamine were greatly improved by the anodization, producing peak currents nearly 20 times higher than un-

Microelectrodes   107

treated fibers. Some fibers were treated in reverse order, first by anodization, then by vacuum heat treatment. In this case, Swain and Kuwana (1992), found that the carbon surface could be annealed to remove the anodic-produced surface fractures. Furthermore, these fibers had lower capacitances than the untreated fibers that had received only vacuum heat treatment. They concluded that vacuum heat treatment can be used to remove surface irregularities on the carbon fibers.

5.1.16 Laser Modified Carbon Surfaces

Strein and Ewing (1991) found that carbon fiber microelectrodes had improved charge transfer properties after pulsing the tip with a nitrogen laser. The microelectrode was immersed in water and held at a potential between -0.1 to -0.2 V. Approximately 140 pulses of three-nanosecond duration were applied over a seven second period. Current was measured to confirm that the laser pulse was hitting the tip. Presumably, the laser energy vaporized surface oxides and may have exposed more reactive sites. Carbon fiber microelectrodes treated in this manner could reduce dopamine at a lower potential, and the reversibility of the cyclic scan wave was found to be less dependent on pH.

5.1.17 Measurement Requirements

High-impedance electrometers and carefully shielded circuits are required to use microelectrodes and take advantage of the rapidity of their responses. Positive feedback capacitance neutralization can be used to reduce the capacitance of some types of microelectrodes used in potentiometric measurements. Many researchers have found that the electrical properties change as the microelectrode is covered with a greater depth of liquid. Often electromagnetic noise and vibration can be a problem, requiring a shielded metal cage around the measuring apparatus which is mounted on a vibration isolation table.

5.1.18 Electrical Shielding

Techniques for improved electrical shielding include physically surrounding the microelectrode with the reference. Microelectrodes have been coated with conductive silver paint, or by metal vapor deposition (sputtering). Kottra and Frömpter (1982) described two techniques for shielding glass micropipettes. When they coated the outer surface of the microelectrode with silver which was then insulated with a polymer coat, they found large capacitive loads between the microelectrode and the shield. This was due to the physical contact between the shield and the bath solution. As a second design, a double-concentric microelectrode was made, with the externally coated microelectrode at the center. The outer microelectrode was filled with either Sylgard or polystyrol lacquer to seal the two microelectrodes together and insulate the tips. This design was found to reduce the capacitive load significantly, since the shield was not in contact with the bath solution.

Nair et al. (1980) also coated the external surface of PO_2 microelectrodes with silver using metal vapor sputtering in vacuum. The external Ag/AgCl coating could be used as a reference anode. They also plated iron on the outside of the tip, which could be electrodeposited into tissue for later histological identification of the measurement site using an appropriate stain. This technique was used to confirm which type of cells the microelectrode had taken measurements from in the cat carotid body.

5.1.19 Clinical Measurements with Microelectrodes

There have been some limited clinical applications using etched metal microelectrodes for measuring tissue PO_2 in human tissues. Ehrly (1990) has reviewed his measurements of human muscle tissue PO_2 made in German hospitals. Microelectrodes were inserted into muscles in the lower limbs of patients with intermittent claudication. The tissue PO_2 was found to be lower than similar muscle tissue measurements from a control group of healthy volunteers. Measurements have been made in resting and exercising muscles. The beneficial effects of various drug treatments (buflomedil, calciumdobesilate, pentoxyfylline, and urokinase) on increasing muscle tissue PO_2 in intermittent claudication patients were also reviewed. In another application, Sakaue et al. (1989) used a small polarographic O_2 electrode during vitreous surgery to measure the aqueous humor O_2 tension in the human eye. Austin et al. (1977) used a 25 μm diameter, Teflon-coated platinum wire "microelectrode" to measure brain tissue PO_2 at a depth of approximately 2 mm in the human cortex. This size may be somewhat large to be considered as a true microelectrode, and absolute PO_2 values were not calculated. An optical measurement of cytochrome a,a_3 reduction was also obtained at 605 nm relative to a reference wavelength at 590 nm. They showed that brain tissue PO_2 levels were improved after microsurgery to create anastomoses from the superficial temporal artery in patients with symptoms of transient ischemic episodes or with incomplete strokes.

5.2 ENZYME MODIFIED MICROELECTRODES

There has been relatively little research into developing enzyme modified biosensors with true microelectrode dimensions. Silver (1980) briefly described a glucose microbiosensor constructed from an etched platinum-iridium wire microelectrode with a 1 μm tip. The tip was flashed with platinum black, treated with glucose oxidase, and coated with a cellulose diacetate membrane. Glucose measurements were made in rat brains. A very small fall in glucose from 2.8 to 2.6 mM was measured in the rat cerebral cortex when cerebral blood flow was significantly reduced by inflating a cuff around the rat's neck. He reported that glucose fell to zero when the blood flow was completely arrested, but these measurements are probably not very meaningful since the PO_2, which was measured by another microelectrode in some experiments, fell to zero. This type of glucose biosensor would no longer be sensitive in the absence of O_2 [Equation (91)]. His reported measurements of very low glucose levels (<0.4 mM) during incomplete ischemia, when the brain blood flow and tissue PO_2 were very low, are also questionable since the glucose biosensor may have been operating in an O_2-limited range. He reported that brain glucose levels were elevated after releasing occlusion, returning to normal in 15 to 45 minutes. Hyperglycemic rats were also studied. These animals had much longer periods of elevated brain glucose levels after restoring blood flow, lasting for two to three hours.

5.2.1 Co-Deposited Glucose Oxidase and Rhodium

Wang and Angnes (1992) co-deposited rhodium and glucose oxidase on a carbon fiber microelectrode using a single electroplating step. Rhodium was added (100 ppm concentration) to a solution containing glucose oxidase solution, and was plated at -0.8 V in a stirred solution for 10 min at pH 4.5. The resulting electrodeposited material on the carbon fiber surface was observed under scanning electron microscopy and was found to be very rough. This type of microelectrode would probably not be useful for insertion into tissues, since the surface coating is not likely to remain attached to the carbon fiber.

5.2.2 Recessed Glucose Microbiosensors

A recessed carbon fiber glucose microbiosensor design has been recently described by Kawagoe et al. (1991a, 1991b). The 7 μm carbon fiber was sealed with epoxy into a glass capillary and the tip ground on a micropipette beveler. The total tip diameter was about 20 μm. The carbon fiber was electrochemically etched away in 0.5 mM potassium dichromate and 5 M sulfuric acid using a 20 V peak-to-peak sine wave at 60 Hz. This created a cone-shaped tip, recessed back from the opening of the glass tip by about 10 to 40 μm. For use as an electron conductor, organic salt crystals of tetra-thiafulvalene-tetracyanoquinodimethane were electrochemically deposited into the recess at a current of 0.13 μA. Glucose oxidase was introduced into the remaining recess by dipping the tip into an 80 μL volume of aqueous buffer containing 5 mg (750 U) of the enzyme. Glucose oxidase was cross-linked by adding 3 μL of 25% aqueous glutaraldehyde to the buffer. This was found to permit higher current densities and less drift than carbon microelectrodes where the enzyme was simply adsorbed onto the surface. The apparent Michaelis-Menten constant (K_m) for the enzyme-catalyzed reaction was determined to be around 14 mM. This is consistent with earlier K_m evaluations for glucose oxidase.

Some of the glucose microbiosensors were also treated with glutaraldehyde cross-linked ascorbate oxidase [EC 1.10.3.3]. The rationale for this treatment was for the possible minimization of interference from ascorbate since the reaction

$$\text{ascorbate oxidase}$$

$$2\text{L-ascorbate} + O_2 \rightarrow 2\text{dehydroascorbate} + 2H_2O \qquad (111)$$

takes place when O_2 is present. Cyclic voltammograms relative to a saturated calomel electrode were measured for various conditions. The glucose microbiosensors had an initial sensitivity loss of about 20% during the first hour of operation, then they stabilized and could be used for several hours. The 90% response time to a change in glucose was < 1.5 sec. The current was not sensitive to flow changes in the range from 0.25 to 1 mL/min. The electron transfer through the conducting salt was still competing with O_2 as an electron source. Oxygen was found to be less of a source of interference for the glucose microbiosensor at higher potentials and at higher glucose concentrations. The O_2 interference was found to be less than reported for some previous glucose biosensors in the literature. The microbiosensors treated with ascorbate oxidase were tested for glucose sensitivity in the presence of 300 μM ascorbate. The current response to 1 mM glucose was larger by about 1.9 times. Although the ascorbate interference was reduced, the ascorbate oxidase/glucose oxidase microbiosensors were still sensitive to O_2. Uric acid was also tested and no significant interference was found.

5.2.3 Acetylcholine Microbiosensors

Microbiosensors for detecting acetylcholine were also fabricated by Kawagoe et al. (1991a), by introducing 125 U acetylcholine esterase [EC 3.1.1.7] and 125 U choline oxidase [EC 1.1.3.17] into the etched carbon fiber recess and cross-linking the enzyme with glutaraldehyde. The enzymes catalyze the following series of reactions

acetylcholine esterase

acetylcholine $+$ H_2O $\rightarrow$ acetate $+$ choline

choline oxidase

choline $+$ O_2 $\rightarrow$ betain aldehyde $+$ H_2O_2

choline oxidase

betain aldehyde $+$ H_2O $\rightarrow$ betain $+$ H_2O_2

(112)

in the presence of O_2. The microelectrodes were also treated with the organic salt tetrathiafulvalene-tetracyanoquinodimethane as the electron donor in the last two reaction steps instead of O_2. The apparent Michaelis-Menten constant (K_m) for the enzyme-catalyzed reaction was determined and found to be consistent with earlier estimations. The 90% response time for these microbiosensors was <4 seconds. Unlike the O_2-limited behavior of glucose microbiosensors at low glucose levels, O_2 was found to be less of an interfering factor at low acetylcholine concentrations. However, the acetylcholine microbiosensors were also sensitive to ascorbate, which could cause significant interference for measurements in tissues where low acetylcholine levels are expected. An earlier glass microelectrode modified with immobilized acetylcholinesterase for detecting acetylcholine was described by Suaud-Chagny and Pujol (1985). When a phosphate buffer at pH $=$ 8 was used for the potential measurement, a lower detection limit of 10^{-5} M was achieved.

None of the microbiosensors fabricated by Kawagoe et al. (1991a, 1991b) described previously were tested in tissue, but the recessed design, with the enzymes contained within the recess, should be superior to microbiosensors with enzyme-coated tips. The surface coating on the latter design may be more easily removed during insertion and movement through tissues.

5.3 MINIATURIZED ARRAYS

Many of the same advantages for microelectrodes can be achieved with miniaturized arrays, overcoming the disadvantage of needing to amplify very small currents when amperometric measurements are made. The beneficial effect of miniaturizing an electrochemical transducer by forming an array of microcathodes is illustrated in Figure 5.3. For a single cathode, there can be significant depletion of the analyte from the sample (right panel) near the transducer surface due to the electrochemical reactions. If the boundary layer extends out into a flowing sample, there could be significant measurement errors due to convective disturbances. This may be troublesome with electrochemical transducers used in flow injection analysis techniques. The effective distance for this boundary layer would depend on the analyte concentration, with higher concentrations creating greater depletion effects. If the same surface area is available for the electrochemical reaction using a miniaturized array, there will be less disturbance of the analyte concentration around the biosensor, as illustrated in the left panel. The same current should be measured for an array as for a single cathode with an equivalent area. However, there can be complications if the microcathodes are spaced too closely together. Localized depletion effects

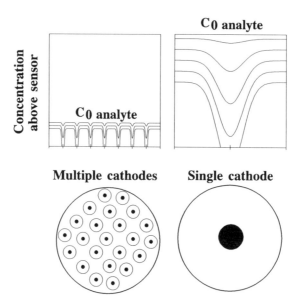

FIGURE 5.3. *With multiple cathodes there is less disturbance of concentration field near an electrochemical transducer compared to a single cathode with the same total area.*

could occur, especially at higher analyte concentrations, interacting with each microcathode.

5.3.1 O_2 Electrodes

The multiarray approach has been successfully used for O_2 electrodes. Kessler and Grunwald (1969) developed a multiwire surface O_2 electrode that was subsequently used in numerous animal experiments by Kessler and others. Both bare cathode and membrane-covered designs have been used. The individual currents, usually from eight symmetrically spaced, 15 μm diameter Pt cathodes, were monitored. Frequency distribution histograms have been generated for the tissue PO_2 values measured on the various organ surfaces that have been studied. This type of multiarray surface PO_2 electrode was used clinically on human leg skeletal muscles by Schönleben et al. (1978) to monitor tissue PO_2 in critically ill patients during various maneuvers including blood transfusion and administration of sodium nitroprusside to control blood pressure. Sinagowitz et al. (1978) used a similar multiarray surface PO_2 electrode to measure renal tissue PO_2 in patients with diseased kidneys, and followed tissue PO_2 after restoring blood flow to transplanted donor kidneys in three patients. The multiarray O_2 electrodes were gas sterilized for these clinical studies.

Whalen and Spande (1980) developed a multiarray O_2 electrode with 10 to 20 glass-coated 5 to 10 μm diameter gold wire cathodes sealed with epoxy in a small (23 gauge) hypodermic needle that could be inserted into tissue. The gold was recessed back into the glass coating by electrochemical etching. The combined current from the recessed microcathode array was measured for this application. The stainless steel hypodermic needle housing the array could be used as a reference anode without excessive drift.

Whalen and Buerk (unpublished) used a hypodermic needle PO_2 electrode in a clinical setting to evaluate whether heart tissue PO_2 levels were improved after bypass surgery. Only one patient was studied. No improvement in tissue PO_2 was seen, and the patient subsequently died during postoperative recovery. Similar needle-type electrodes have been used clinically in several German hospitals, although usually these electrodes were designed with a single, unrecessed cathode. For example, Fleckenstein et al. (1984) measured muscle PO_2 in healthy volunteers and in critically ill patients, and demonstrated that dopamine infusions could increase the tissue PO_2.

5.3.2 Transparent O_2 Electrode Array

Sargent and Gough (1991) designed a transparent O_2 electrode array consisting of eight Pt working electrodes with diameters around 100 μm and spaced 200 μm apart, with a larger common Ag/AgCl reference electrode and a larger Pt counterelectrode. All of the electrodes were made by semiconductor photolithographic methods. Glass was used as the support structure for the device. A thin layer of polyimide was spin coated on the glass and cured by UV light at high temperature, then Pt was sputtered to form a uniform, approximately 370 Å thick metal layer. The electrochemical transducers, bonding pads, and electrical connection lines were formed by standard photoresist methods. Metal was etched away in an acid bath and the photoresist was removed by washing in organic solvents.

A similar sputtering and photoresist technique was used to make the Ag/AgCl reference electrode pattern. A lift-off method was also tried, but the reference electrode was not as sharply defined by this fabrication technique. After the final pattern was made, a 20 μm thick layer of polyimide was applied as an electrical insulator. Two membranes were applied in the final steps. First, a 10 μm thick layer of poly(hydroxyethylmethacrylate) dissolved in methanol was spin coated over the electrodes. After drying, this membrane was allowed to soak in an electrolyte solution. A final silicone rubber membrane was spin coated to a thickness of around 30 to 100 μm. The device was bench tested and also used to make physiological PO_2 measurements on the surface of a surgically exposed rate cremaster muscle preparation. The individual O_2 transducer currents were monitored. The transparent materials used for this sensor design allow the underlying microcirculation to be observed through the device, although this was not done in their preliminary research.

5.3.3 Band Arrays

Samuelsson et al. (1991) describe a photolithographic and ion beam etching method for fabricating a microarray with bands of ultramicroelectrodes. They used conventional photoresist pattern techniques to produce bands of gold, approximately 1 μm wide and 200 nm thick, on SiO_2 substrate. The spacing between bands was varied for different photoresist patterns to create repeated spacing of either 10, 100, or 1,000 μm between bands. The gold bands were covered with Si_3N_4 insulation. The bands were then trimmed by reactive ion beam etching down to the SiO_2 substrate, leaving very thin (200 nm) and sharply defined strips of gold exposed at each vertical edge of the etched channel. The wider horizontal band of gold was still covered with insulation. These microarrays were found to have better signal-to-background noise ratios, and reduced double layer capacitances compared to the untrimmed, larger band arrays produced by the photoresist pattern. Diffusional overlap effects were seen with the closest (10 μm) spacing pattern between bands.

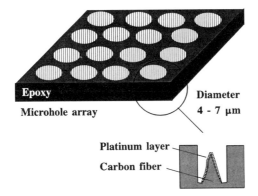

FIGURE 5.4. *Microhole array made from epoxy-carbon material with recessed platinized carbon fiber cathodes for O_2 measurements, designed by Morita and Shimuzu (1989).*

5.3.4 Microhole Arrays

A recessed microhole array of carbon fibers in epoxy has been fabricated and tested by Morita and Shimizu (1989), which is shown schematically in Figure 5.4. A bundle of 1,000 carbon fibers with 7 μm diameters were heat treated at 2,000°C and then impregnated with epoxy resin. After drying at 130°C, a rod of fibers was cast in epoxy inside a 2 mm diameter polyethylene tube. After curing, sections of the tubing were cut. One end was polished by mechanical abrasion and the other end electrically connected by conductive silver paint. The polished end was immersed in 2 mM sulfuric acid and 0.2 mM sodium sulfate and electrolytically etched at a constant current > 800 mA/cm². Maximum etching depths of around 500 μm could be achieved. After cleaning the etching solution, the carbon fibers were left polarized at − 0.6 versus a saturated calomel reference electrode for an hour, then were electroplated with platinum. A uniform, 0.5 μm platinum layer was produced, based on electron microscopy. The properties of this recessed microarray for use as an O_2 transducer were tested. The current and flow sensitivity were reduced as the recess depth was increased, as expected.

5.3.5 Microporous Array

Another type of microarray was investigated by Cheng et al. (1989), who filled the pores of commercially produced polycarbonate film membranes with carbon particle paste. Pore sizes for different membranes were nominally reported to be 12, 8, and 3 μm by the manufacturer (Nucleopore Corp.). Electron microscopy confirmed the pore diameters, and determined that the pore densities were 6.4×10^4, 8.8×10^4, and 1.36×10^5 pores/cm^2 respectively for each grade of membrane. The pore density information was more accurate than that supplied by the manufacturer, although not markedly different. After filling the pores with carbon paste, the membranes were placed over a larger carbon paste electrode and cyclic voltammograms were measured in Fe(bpy)$_3$(ClO$_4$)$_2$ and K$_2$SO$_4$ solutions relative to an Ag/AgCl reference. Their electrochemical measurements were consistent with the geometrical information with regard to the pore density of the membranes.

Three limiting cases based on theoretical expectations were investigated. At very high scan rates, the diffusion effects should be limited to the immediate vicinity of the pore, with no interactions with other pores. At slower scan rates, diffusion fields should extend out radially from the pore. If the spacing between pores is large enough, there should be no diffusional interactions between pores. At very slow rates, the diffusional fields will overlap. Cheng et al. (1989) confirmed that the microporous array electrode behaved as expected. With the smallest pore diameters (3 μm), evidence for diffusional overlap was found, with estimated distances of only 4.6 μm between pores. The scan rate of their instrument was not fast enough to examine the first limiting case with the smallest pores since they were so closely spaced. In practice, the operating scan rate for the optimum range with minimal diffusional interactions may be difficult to achieve. Furthermore, the pore density of the membranes cannot be manipulated to produce the best microarray. However, it may be possible to minimize interactions by exploiting diffusional limitations if the pores can be partially filled, leaving recesses. This possibility was not investigated.

5.4 SEMICONDUCTOR NEEDLE

Ottosensors Corporation (Cleveland, OH) makes a needle-type probe using thin-film and solid-state fabrication techniques that can have multiple transducers, similar to the device shown schematically in Figure 5.5. Prohaska (1987) described the basic fabrication methods. Needle probes were constructed on a clean, 100 μm thick glass needle substrate, evaporation coated with a 0.1 μm thick triple metal layer. First a thin chromium (Cr) base coat was made to increase adhesion to the glass, then gold was deposited, followed by another layer of Cr. Using photolithographic techniques, a photosensitive insulator layer was deposited and exposed to UV light through a mask designed for a specific multisensor layout. Up to sixteen

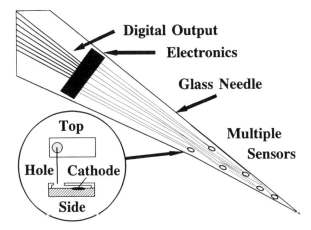

FIGURE 5.5. *Schematic of a glass needle probe with multiple sensors fabricated by photolithographic technology. Signals from each sensor might be amplified with electronic chips fabricated on the device, or processed later through connections at the end.*

transducers can be arranged in a row, spaced 100 μm apart. The metal layer was etched away, leaving the necessary interconnecting pathways from each transducer to bonding pad areas at the upper end of the probe. A second photolithographic step covered the interconnecting pathways with photoresist, leaving the transducers and bonding pads uncovered. For some of the transducers, a 2–3 μm thick layer of silicon nitride (Si_3N_4) insulation was coated over the site by high-energy plasma vapor deposition. The transducer sites can be made very small with appropriate etching techniques, and other metals can be electroplated onto their surfaces.

Presently, needle probes are commercially available with transducers for temperature, biopotential, and O_2 measurements, in combinations or with a single transducer type. The signals are amplified by external electronics, and the probe is suitable for measurements in brain tissue or other biological media. Biopotential recordings can be made from Ag/AgCl electrodes with either small (10 $\times$ 10 μm) or large (50 $\times$ 50 μm) areas. The electrodes are electrolytically plated to form a 1 μm thick silver layer, which is then chlorided by electrolysis in a 1% NaCl solution. For the O_2 transducer, shown schematically in the inset of Figure 5.5, a chamber of 3 μm thick Si_3N_4 is made over the O_2 transducer by plasma vapor deposition. The chamber is roughly 45 μm wide and 80 μm long. Afterwards, a small, 15 μm diameter hole is made in the chamber to provide access to the 25 μm^2 Au electrode. A 1,600 μm^2 Ag/AgCl reference electrode is fabricated nearby. The temperature transducer dimensions are 110 $\times$ 140 μm, using a germanium semiconductor thermistor. The thermistor has a constant 0.5 V applied to it and the resulting current fluctuations are measured as the resistance varies with changes in temperature. As this technology is further developed, eventually all of the required electronics for signal amplification and processing for each transducer channel could be fabricated on the same glass needle. This type of needle probe could also be modified to function as a biosensor by applying suitable enzymes and membranes to the O_2 or potential transducers.

5.5 ENFET BIOSENSORS

The basic operational principle for the field effect transistor (FET) is its ability to vary the resistance of the current path between the source and drain when an electrical field (voltage) is applied to the gate. The semiconductor properties at the source, gate, and drain are determined by traces of impurities such as boron or phosphorus used for doping the SiO_2 substrate, which is normally an insulator. Photolithographic techniques have been developed to fabricate ion-sensitive field effect transistors (ISFET) and metal-oxide semiconductor field effect transistors (MOSFET). These transducers can be further modified for use as enzyme-based biosensors (ENFET).

5.5.1 ISFET

For the ISFET, an ion-selective membrane is placed over the gate and a voltage is applied through an Ag/AgCl or SCE reference in the sample solution. As the ionic concentration varies, the resulting change in electrical field at the gate modulates the conductance of the semiconductor. Ion-sensitive membranes for pH have been made using silicon nitride (Si_3N_4), alumina (Al_2O_3), zirconium oxide (ZrO_2), and tantalum oxide (Ta_2O_5). As discussed previously (Chapter 3), complications can result when there is the possibility for multiple hydrated forms on the metal oxide [Equation (58)]. CO_2 can be sensed by ISFETs using pH changes based on the same principle for electrochemical detection discussed previously (Chapter 3). In addition to H^+ ions, ISFETs with ion-sensitive membranes have also been developed for Na^+, K^+, Ca^{2+}, NH_4^+, Ag^+, Cl^-, and Br^-.

5.5.2 MOSFET

The gate can be fabricated with a metal oxide surface, such as Pt or Pd, which can then serve as a catalyst for different chemical reactions. Gases and chemical vapors can be detected by the transducer, although water vapor can be a significant interfering factor.

5.5.3 ENFET

Either type of semiconductor FET can be modified by placing specific enzymes over the transducer. As discussed previously for the glucose biosensor (Chapter 4), it is often convenient to have a differential sensor with an unmodified transducer to correct for the background conditions that are superimposed on the enzyme modified transducer. A schematic drawing for a urea ENFET using the differential pH measurement technique described by Kurimaya and Kimura (1989, 1991) is shown in Figure 5.6. They deposited a thin layer of thermally oxidized silicon (SiO_2) on a sapphire substrate approximately 350 μm thick. Boron was ion-implanted into the SiO_2 and phosphorus was ion-implanted into the source and drain. They also implanted a small amount of phosphorus into the gate to control the threshold voltage for the FET. The pH sensitivity was achieved by coating a 1,000 μm layer of Si_3N_4 over the two FETs. A 1 μm layer of Au was sputtered for electrical connections.

5.6 ENCAPSULATION AND MEMBRANES

It is imperative that semiconductor devices and the connecting wires that will be immersed in aqueous samples retain their electrical isolation from the sample. For the device just described, Kurimaya and Kimura (1989, 1991) chose sapphire for the bonding substrate and report that it has ex-

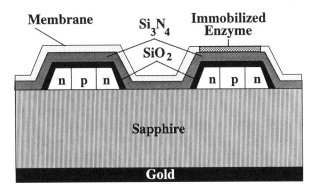

FIGURE 5.6. *Schematic drawing of a differential FET-type biosensor produced by photolithography which uses enzyme modified membranes.*

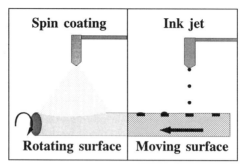

Spin coating	Ink jet
Rotating surface	Moving surface

FIGURE 5.7. *Two methods for applying thin membranes to biosensors. For the spin-coating method, a fine mist is sprayed as the device rotates at 1,000 to 2,000 rpm. With an ink jet, automation methods can be used to apply a small volume at a specific location.*

cellent resistance to water infiltration, allowing it to retain electrical insulation from aqueous samples for long periods. Also, they report that it is not necessary to reinsulate cut edges after separating an individual sensor from a larger wafer. Various types of application methods, ranging from simple dipping followed by solvent evaporation, have been tested by various research groups throughout the world. Spin coating, such as that shown schematically in Figure 5.7, can be used to apply thin membranes. The individual biosensor or a wafer can be coated with different layers, and various techniques can be used to remove the coating if necessary over specific parts of the design. Biomembranes can also be applied over the electrochemical transducer. Special precautions must be taken to apply biomembranes so that they retain their enzymatic activity. An ink jet method, shown schematically in Figure 5.7 (right panel) was developed by Kimura et al. (1988). This method would be especially useful for fabricating biosensors that use expensive enzymes. Automation techniques such as those already in place in the microelectronics industries can be readily adapted to mass production of specialized biosensors. New techniques to attach proteins, or newly engineered proteins (antibodies), and new combinations of enzymes are continuing to be developed in different laboratories.

5.7 REFERENCES

Abatti, P. J. and T. Moriizumi. 1992. "Development of a New Geometrical Form of Micropipette: Electrical Characteristics and an Application as a Potassium Ion Selective Electrode," *IEEE Trans. Biomed. Eng.*, 39:43–48.

Ammann, D. 1986. *Ion-Selective Micro-Electrodes. Principles, Design and Application.* New York, NY: Springer-Verlag.

Austin, G., G. Haugen and J. LaManna. 1977. "Cortical Oxidative Metabolism following Microanastomosis for Brain Ischemia," in *Oxygen and Physiological Function*, F. F. Jöbsis, ed., Dallas, TX: Prof. Inform. Library, pp. 531–544.

Barret, J. and D. G. Whitlock. 1973. "Technique for Beveling Glass Microelectrodes," in *Intracellular Staining in Neurobiology*, S. B. Kater and C. Nicholson, eds., New York, NY: Springer-Verlag.

Brown, K. T. and D. G. Flaming. 1974. "Beveling of Fine Micropipette Electrodes by a Rapid Precision Method," *Science*, 185:693–695.

Brown, K. T. and D. G. Flaming. 1986. *Advanced Micropipette Techniques for Cell Physiology*. New York, NY: J. Wiley and Sons.

Caldwell, P. C. 1956. "Intracellular pH," *Int. Rev. Cytol.*, 5:229–227.

Cheng, I. F., L. D. Whitely and C. R. Martin. 1989. "Ultramicroelectrode Ensembles. Comparison of Experimental and Theoretical Responses and Evaluation of Electroanalytical Detection Limits," *Anal. Chem.*, 61:762–766.

Coury, L. A., Jr., E. W. Huber and W. R. Heineman. 1989. "Applications of Modified Electrodes in the Voltammetric Determination of Catecholamine Neurotransmitters," in *Applied Biosensors*, D. L. Wise, ed., Boston, MA: Butterworths, pp. 1–37.

DeHemptinne, A. 1980. "Intracellular pH and Surface pH in Skeletal and Cardiac Muscle Measured with a Double-Barrelled pH Microelectrode," *Pflüg. Arch.*, 386:121–126.

Ehrly, A. M. 1990. "Pathophysiology of Impaired Oxygen Delivery to Tissue and Associated Medical Problems," in *Drugs and the Delivery of Oxygen to Tissue*, J. S. Fleming, ed., Boca Raton, FL: C.R.C. Press, pp. 1–13.

Fleckenstein, W., K. Reinhart, T. Kersting, R. Dennhardt, A. Jasper, C. Weiss and K. Eyrich. 1984. "Dopamine Effects on the Oxygenation of Human Skeletal Muscle," in *Oxygen Transport to Tissue—VI*, D. Bruley, H. I. Bicher and D. Reneau, eds., New York, NY: Plenum Press; *Adv. Exp. Med. & Biol.*, 180:609–622.

Fry, D. M. 1975. "A Scanning Electron Microscope Method for the Examination of Glass Microelectrode Tips Either Before or After Use," *Experientia*, 31:695.

Hinke, J. A. M. 1967. "Cation-Selective Microelectrodes for Intracellular Use," in *Glass Electrodes for Hydrogen and Other Cations. Principles and Practice*, G. Eisenman, ed., New York, NY: M. Dekker, Inc., pp. 464–477.

Javaheri, S., A. DeHemptinne and I. Leusen. 1984. "Single-Unit pH-Sensitive Double-Barreled Microelectrodes for Extracellular Use," *J. Appl. Physiol.*, 57:907–912.

Kawagoe, J. L., D. E. Niehaus and R. M. Wightman. 1991a. "Enzyme-Modified Organic Conducting Salt Microelectrode," *Anal. Chem.*, 63:2961–2965.

Kawagoe, K. T., J. A. Jankowski and R. M. Wightman. 1991b. "Etched Carbon-Fiber Electrodes as Amperometric Detectors of Catecholamine Secretion from Isolated Biological Cells," *Anal. Chem.*, 63:1589–1593.

Kessler, M. and W. Grunwald. 1969. "Possibilities of Measuring Oxygen Pressure Fields in Tissue by Multiwire Platinum Electrodes," in *International Symposium on Oxygen Pressure Recording*. New York, NY: Karger, p. 147.

Kiani, M. F. and R. W. Schubert. 1988. "Oxygen Sensitivity of Recessed and Unrecessed Antimony pH Microlectrodes," *Med. & Biol. Eng. & Comp.*, 26:541–546.

Kimura, J., Y. Kawana and T. Kuriyama. 1988. "An Immobilized Enzyme Membrane Fabrication Method Using an Ink Jet Nozzle," *Biosensors*, 4:41–52.

Kottra, G. and E. Frömter. 1982. "A Simple Method for Constructing Shielded, Low-Capacitance Glass Microelectrodes," *Pflüg. Arch.*, 395:156–158.

Kuriyama, T. and J. Kimura. 1989. "An ISFET Biosensor," in *Applied Biosensors*, D. L. Wise, ed., Boston, MA: Butterworths, pp. 93–114.

Kuriyama, T. and J. Kimura. 1991. "FET-Based Biosensors," in *Biosensor Principles and Applications*, L. J. Blum and P. R. Coulet, eds., New York, NY: M. Dekker, Inc., pp. 139–162.

Lederer, W. J., A. J. Spindler and D. A. Eisner. 1979. "Thick Slurry Beveling," *Pflüg. Arch.*, 381:287–288.

Ling, G. and R. W. Gerard. 1949. "The Normal Membrane Potential of Sartorius Fibers," *J. Cell. Comp. Physiol.*, 34:383–390.

Linsenmeier, R. A. and C. M. Yancey. 1987. "Improved Fabrication of Double-Barreled Recessed Cathode O_2 Microelectrodes," *J. Appl. Physiol.*, 63:2554–2557.

Lissilour, S. and C. Godinot. 1990. "Precise, Easy Measurement of Glass Pipet Tips for Microinjection or Electrophysiology," *Biotech.*, 9:401–404.

Mittman, S., D. G. Flaming, D. R. Copenhagen and J. H. Begum. 1987. "Bubble Pressure Measurement of Micropipette Tip Outer Diameter," *J. Neurosci. Meth.*, 22:161–169.

Morita, K. and Y. Shimizu. 1989. "Microhole Array for Oxygen Electrode," *Anal. Chem.*, 61:159–162.

Nair, P. K., D. G. Buerk and J. H. Halsey, Jr. 1986. "Microregional pH Changes in Ischemic Gerbil Brain," *Fed. Proc.*, 45:1007 (abstract).

Nair, P., J. I. Spande and W. J. Whalen. 1980. Marking the Tip Location of PO_2 Microelectrodes or Glass Micropipettes," *J. Appl. Physiol.*, 49:916–918.

Nair, P. K., J. I. Spande and W. J. Whalen. 1985. "A Microelectrode for Measuring Intracellular pH," in *Oxygen Transport to Tissue—VI*, D. F. Bruley, H. I. Bicher and D. Reneau, eds., New York, NY: Plenum Press; *Adv. Exp. Med. & Biol.*, 180:881–886.

Ogden, T. E., M. C. Citron and R. Pierantoni. 1978. "The Jet Stream Microbeveler: An Inexpensive Way to Bevel Ultrafine Glass Micropipettes," *Science*, 201:469–470.

Penner, R. M., M. J. Heben, T. L. Longin and N. S. Lewis. 1990. "Fabrication and Use of Nanometer-Sized Electrodes in Electrochemistry," *Science Wash. DC*, 250:1118–1121.

Rice, M. E. and C. Nicholson. 1989. "Measurement of Nanomolar Dopamine Diffusion Using Low-Noise Perfluorinated Ionomer Coated Carbon Fiber Microelectrodes and High-Speed Cyclic Voltammetry," *Anal. Chem.*, 61:1805–1810.

Prohaska, O. 1987. "Thin-Film Micro-Electrodes for *in vivo* Electrochemical Analysis," in *Biosensors, Fundamentals and Applications*, A. P. F. Turner, I. Karube and G. S. Wilson, NY: Oxford Univ. Press, pp. 377–389.

Samuelsson, M., M. Armgarth and C. Nylander. 1991. "Microstep Electrodes: Band Ultramicroelectrodes Fabricated by Photolithography and Reactive Ion Etching," *Anal. Chem.*, 63:931–936.

Sargent, B. J. and D. A. Gough. 1991. "Design and Validation of the Transparent Oxygen Sensor Array," *IEEE Trans. Biomed. Eng.*, 38:476–482.

Sakaue, H., Y. Tsukahara, A. Negi, N. Ogino and Y. Honda. 1989. "Measurement of Vitreous Oxygen Tension in Human Eyes," *Jpn. J. Ophthalmol.*, 33:199–203.

Satake, N., Y. Matsumura and M. Fujimoto. 1980. "Temperature Coefficient of and Oxygen Effect on the Antimony Microelectrode," *Jap. J. Physiol.*, 30:671–687.

Schönleben, K., J. P. Hauss, U. Spiegel, H. Bünte and M. Kessler. 1978. "Monitoring of Tissue PO_2 in Patients during Intensive Care," in *Oxygen Transport to Tissue—III*, I. A. Silver, M. Erecińska and H. I. Bicher, eds., New York, NY: Plenum Press; *Adv. Exp. Med. & Biol.*, 94:593–598.

Silver, I. A. 1980. "Oxygen, pH and Glucose Measurements in Cerebral Ischaemia," in *Advances in Physiological Sciences, Volume 25: Oxygen Transport to Tissue*, A. G. B. Kovach, E. Dóra, M. Kessler and I. A. Silver, eds., Budapest, Hungary: Pergamon Press, pp. 103–104.

Sinagowitz, E., M. Golsong and J. J. Halbfaß. 1978. "Local Tissue PO_2 in Kidney Surgery and Transplantation," in *Oxygen Transport to Tissue—III*, I. A. Silver, M. Erecińska and H. I. Bicher, eds., New York, NY: Plenum Press; *Adv. Exp. Med. & Biol.*, 94:721–727.

Strein, T. G. and A. G. Ewing. 1991. "*In situ* Laser Activation of Carbon Fiber Microdisk Electrodes," *Anal. Chem.*, 63:194–198.

Suaud-Chagny, M. F. and J. F. Pujol. 1985. "Enzyme Microelectrode for Acetylcholine Detection," *Analysis*, 13:25.

Swain, G. M. and T. Kuwana. 1992. "Anodic Fracturing and Vacuum Heat Treated Annealing of Pitch-Based Carbon Fibers," *Anal. Chem.*, 64:565–568.

Thomas, R. C. 1974. "Intracellular pH of Snail Neurones Measured with a New pH-Sensitive Glass Microelectrode," *J. Physiol. London*, 238:159–180.

Tsacopoulos, M. and A. Lehmenkühler. 1977. "A Double-Barrelled Pt-Microelectrode for Simultaneous Measurement of PO_2 and Bioelectrical Activity in Excitable Tissues," *Experientia*, 33:1337–1338.

Vieira, F. L. and G. Malnic. 1968. "Hydrogen Ion Secretion by Rat Renal Cortical Tubules as Studied by an Antimony Microelectrode," *Am. J. Physiol.*, 214:710–718.

Wang, J. and L. Angnes. 1992. "Miniaturized Glucose Sensors Based on Electrochemical Codeposition of Rhodium and Glucose Oxidase onto Carbon-Fiber Electrodes," *Anal. Chem.*, 64:456–459.

Whalen, W. J. and J. I. Spande. 1980. "A Hypodermic Needle PO_2 Electrode," *J. Appl. Physiol.*, 48:186–187.

Whalen, W. J., P. Nair and D. G. Buerk. 1973. "Oxygen Tension in the Beating Cat Heart *in Situ*," in *Oxygen Supply—Theoretical and Practical Aspects of Oxygen Supply and Microcirculation of Tissue*, M. Kessler, D. F. Bruley, L. C. Clark, Jr., D. W. Lübbers, I. A. Silver and J. Strauss, eds., W. Germany: Urban and Schwarzenberg, pp. 199–201.

Whalen, W. J., J. Riley and P. Nair. 1967. "A Microelectrode for Measuring Intracellular PO_2," *J. Appl. Physiol.*, 23:798–801.

Wolbarsht, M. L., E. F. MacNichol and H. G. Wagner. 1960. "Glass Insulated Platinum Microelectrode," *Science Wash. DC*, 132:1309–1310.

CHAPTER 6

Optical Technology

There have been many different optical technologies that have become vital components of modern biochemical and chemical analytical instrumentation. Most of these technologies have also been modified for use as optical transducers in biosensors. The basic theory and some specific applications for various types of optical biosensors are described in the following section.

6.1 PRINCIPLES OF OPTICAL MEASUREMENTS

6.1.1 Measuring Light

Light intensity (the number of photons observed per unit time) can be measured by extremely sensitive photomultiplier devices with excellent accuracy. The light coming from a source may either be transmitted through or reflected back from the sample. The output signal from photomultiplier tube detectors can be further amplified using conventional electronic circuitry without adding significant noise. However, photomultiplier tubes are not able to perform as well at light wavelengths above 1 μm. Silicon photodiodes, which have lower internal resistances and have inherently more electrical noise, are roughly 1,000 times less sensitive. Nonetheless, silicon photodiodes may still have sufficient gain for applications where less precise measurements are required. Silicon photodiodes are also less expensive and more rugged than photomultiplier tubes and are definitely more useful for portable instrumentation.

Intermediate characteristics are now available with silicon avalanche photodiodes. Although they still have more internal noise than photomul-

125

tipliers, silicon avalanche photodiodes can have excellent gain, especially when operated at lower temperatures. Low-cost plastic fiberoptics or other optical waveguides can be used to direct and pick up light to all three types of light detectors, as will be discussed later in this chapter. Silicon avalanche photodiodes may be more useful for fiberoptics applications where a smaller detection area is needed.

Excellent optical filters are available for instruments where a specific light wavelength needs to be monitored. Well-regulated light sources are also available for applications where a reference signal or an excitation signal at a specific light wavelength and pulse duration is required. Mechanical light-chopping systems can also divide light beams into separate reference and measuring beams. In some applications, the background light intensity will affect the overall sensitivity of the optical technique. In other cases, it is the rate of light intensity change that determines the sensitivity of the measurement. There are four basic operational principles for biosensors using optical technology: absorption and reflection spectroscopy, chemiluminescence, fluorescence, and phosphorescence.

6.2 ABSORPTION SPECTROSCOPY

6.2.1 Basic Theory

The Lambert-Beer Law is used to characterize the intensity of transmitted light (I) through a uniform medium as a function of the incident light (I_0) when the optical properties are affected by the chemical concentration (C). The intensity is given by

$$I = I_0 \exp^{-\epsilon C \Delta x} \qquad (113)$$

where ϵ is the extinction coefficient and Δx is the thickness of the medium. Light scattering in the sample is not considered. The optical density of the medium, defined as

$$\text{O.D.} = \ln\left(\frac{I_0}{I}\right) \qquad (114)$$

can change as the concentrations of different chemical species vary in the medium. A spectrum of light will be absorbed in some range of wavelengths, which would be distinct for each chemical species. Variations in light absorption are due to the vibrational and rotational movements for different chemical bonds in the molecules in the light path which absorb energy at different wavelengths.

Usually, a light intensity signal in the presence of a chemical species (I_C) is compared to a reference signal (I_R) which is measured when there is no chemical species present ($C = 0$) or at some other calibration level at a known concentration ($C = C_0$). Concentration can be monitored by comparing light spectrum changes with the reference spectrum. This comparison is usually nonlinear. The measured concentration might be related to light intensities by a power law

$$C_{\text{measured}} = a + b\left(\frac{I_C}{I_R}\right)^n \tag{115}$$

or by a power series,

$$C_{\text{measured}} = a + b\left(\frac{I_C}{I_R}\right) + c\left(\frac{I_C}{I_R}\right)^2 + \dots \tag{116}$$

where a, b, and c are empirically determined constants, or by some other nonlinear mathematical relationship.

6.2.2 Interpreting Light Signals

The principle of light absorption spectroscopy measurements is illustrated in Figure 6.1. In the bottom panel, several light absorption curves

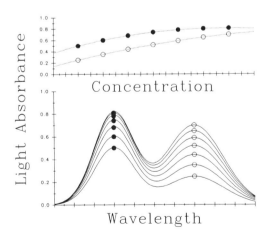

FIGURE 6.1. *Example of change in light absorbance with concentration of a chemical substrate. In this case, two peaks in light absorbance at two different wavelengths (bottom panel) are observed, which are both related to concentration (top panel).*

are shown for different concentration levels of a chemical species that alters the optical properties of the sample. This hypothetical example has two distinct absorption peaks for the chemical species, and both peaks vary with concentration as shown in the top panel. For this example, a better signal-to-noise ratio would be obtained by monitoring the light absorption for the peak at the higher wavelength (open circles), since it has a relatively greater change in signal with concentration. While the peaks in this example remain at the same light wavelength, in the real world a light absorption peak and the wavelength where it occurs could both shift as the concentration varies. Also, a distinct peak may not always be observed. In this case, it may be possible to pick a suitable wavelength on some other part of the absorption curve that would be useful for monitoring concentration changes.

There are several possible sources of error with the light absorption method, including light scattering and physical limitations for the depth of light penetration that can be achieved with different samples. Care must be taken to minimize internal light reflections from surfaces within the sample chamber or in the optical components. If the measurement is being made in living tissues, the light power cannot be too great, to avoid thermal damage to the cells. Disturbances from external light sources can also influence the measurement. If the sampled region has nonuniform optical properties, or these properties change with time, it may be very difficult to interpret absorbance measurements. Also, water itself has high background absorption which may be problematic for some molecules and in some light wavelength ranges, e.g., in the infrared around 975 nm.

6.3 REFLECTANCE SPECTROSCOPY

There may be advantages to measuring the light reflected back from a surface or from deeper layers of a medium. Changes in the intensity of reflected light may accurately represent physical as well as chemical events that occur. As shown schematically in Figure 6.2, the depth of light that penetrates into an ideal, nonscattering medium is given by

$$\Delta x = \frac{\lambda}{2\pi n_1 \sqrt{\sin^2 \theta - \left(\frac{n_2}{n_1}\right)^2}} \tag{117}$$

when the relative refractive index of the transmission path (n_1) is greater than in the medium ($n_1 > n_2$). When illuminated at an oblique incidence

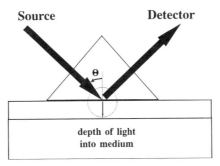

FIGURE 6.2. *Principle of optical reflectance measurement. Light transmitted through the optic fiber or waveguide penetrates into the surface material to a total depth that depends on the difference in refractive indexes.*

angle θ, the incident light is totally reflected. It is possible to have an evanescent wave that only penetrates very short distances ($< 1,000$ Å) into the medium, allowing study of localized surface phenomena. In other applications, it may be desirable to have the light penetrate as deeply as possible into the medium. In complex media, there may be layers with different refractive indexes and coefficients for light absorption and scattering.

6.4 CHEMILUMINESCENCE

6.4.1 Basic Theory

Luminescence is generally defined as the emission of light from atoms or molecules as a result of a transition from an electronically excited state to a lower energy state. Some chemical reactions can create excited intermediates. There are a number of chemiluminescent reagents that can be used to detect specific biochemical reactions that occur, either from isolated test tube studies or directly from living plant and animal cells. In the process of completing these reactions, light is emitted. This phenomenon is often described as "cold light" since photons are released without intermediate formation of heat. No external source of light is required to initiate this reaction, and the whole sample is involved.

A simplified model of chemiluminescence can be represented by two steps (activation and decay)

$$A \xrightarrow{k_1} A' \xrightarrow{k_2} h\nu \tag{118}$$

involving coupled first order reactions, where k_1 is the rate of activation and k_2 is the rate of decay. The light intensity of the emitted signal is then given by

$$I = \text{constant} \cdot k_2 C_A \tag{119}$$

where the scaling constant includes the amplifier gain and other factors associated with the measurement of the light signal. The time-dependent response for the light intensity is given by

$$I = \text{constant} \cdot C_{A_0} \frac{k_1 k_2}{k_2 - k_1} \, (\exp^{-k_1 t} - \exp^{-k_2 t}) \tag{120}$$

where C_{A_0} is the initial concentration of the chemiluminescent substrate. The maximum intensity (I_{max}) of emitted light is reached at the time

$$t_{max} = \frac{\ln (k_2/k_1)}{k_2 - k_1} \tag{121}$$

I_{max} can be found by substituting t_{max} into Equation (120).

Normalized light intensity responses predicted from this simple theory are shown in Figure 6.3. Responses are shown for cases where the decay

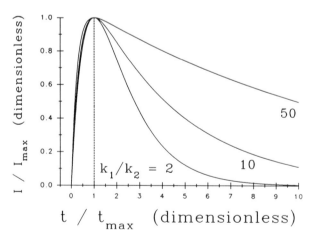

FIGURE 6.3. *Normalized intensities of transient light emission predicted from Equations (120) and (121) for first order activation (k_1) and decay (k_2) as a function of normalized time. Transients are shown for progressively longer decay (smaller k_2) of chemiluminescent signal.*

rate is 2, 10, and 50 times greater than the activation rate, illustrating progressively slower decay times.

6.4.2 Signal Measurements

Since chemiluminescent signals are normally very rapid, the photomultiplier and amplifying electronics must have a suitable bandwidth to faithfully record the event. The actual physical mixing of the substrate into the chemiluminescent reagent must also be very rapid. It is possible to manipulate the chemiluminescence decay rate by either changing the concentration of the enzyme, or by adding inhibitors of the enzyme. If the decay rate is slowed down, as illustrated in Figure 6.3, a quasi–steady state analysis can be made, measuring the peak "glow" (sustained light intensity) of the sample. This type of measurement is also less sensitive to the rate of mixing.

A familiar example of chemiluminescence comes from the firefly (*Photinus pyralis*), which uses the enzyme luciferase [EC 1.13.12.7]. In the presence of Mg^{2+} and the substrate luciferin, ATP is utilized in the following reaction

$$luciferin + ATP + O_2 \rightarrow$$
$$oxyluciferin + AMP + PPi + CO_2 + h\nu \tag{122}$$

catalyzed by luciferase. The light emission is yellow-green with a peak around 560 nm. The quantum yield, i.e., the ratio of the number of photons produced for a given number of molecules, is remarkably high for the firefly system, on the order of 0.9.

A number of synthetic compounds, including luminol, lophine, lucigen, and derivatives of oxalates, emit light in the presence of H_2O_2. For example, luminol reacts as follows

$$luminol + 2H_2O_2 + OH^- \rightarrow$$
$$3\text{-aminophthalate} + N_2 + 3H_2O + h\nu \tag{123}$$

under alkaline conditions with an appropriate catalyst or co-oxidant. This reaction is much less efficient, with a quantum yield around 0.2.

6.5 FLUORESCENCE

6.5.1 Basic Theory

An external source of light is required to initiate fluorescence, which occurs in the material excited by the light source. The fluorescent response is assumed to occur instantaneously with excitation, and the emitted light is also assumed to obey the Lambert-Beer Law. Parker's Law has been used to represent the fluorescent light intensity I_f

$$I_f = \text{constant} \cdot C\epsilon\phi_f\Delta x \qquad (124)$$

from a sample with thickness Δx, where ϵ is the extinction coefficient and ϕ_f is the quantum yield of the fluorescent dye. The energy from the excitation light source must not be destructive to the biological sample or cause bleaching of the fluorescent dye in the sample. Fluorescent imaging systems generally employ pulsed light excitation using lasers or mechanical light-chopping devices. The light emitted is usually much weaker and generally occurs at a longer wavelength than the excitation signal, as illustrated in Figure 6.4. The maximum light intensity of the fluorescent signal and its subsequent decay with time can depend on the concentrations of reactants or co-reactants that are participating in highly specific chemical reactions.

6.5.2 Signal Measurement

One of the major difficulties in interpreting fluorescent measurements is the close proximity of the relatively large excitation signal, which may have multiple peaks at other wavelengths, with the much smaller amplitude

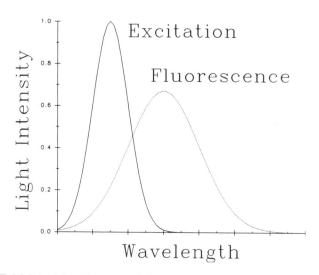

FIGURE 6.4. *Principle of fluorescent light emitted in response to an excitation light signal, with the resulting emission peak of fluorescent light occurring at a different wavelength.*

emission signal, which may also have multiple resonant peaks at other wavelengths. Very small differences may exist between the major wavelength bands, which could be as close together as 30 nm. Newly developed techniques include the use of multiple excitation wavelengths. With confocal microscopy techniques, three-dimensional images of intracellular concentrations using various fluorescent probes are now possible.

In the past, fluorescence measurements have been limited to the UV and visible portions of the spectrum. However, with the development of solid state lasers such as Nd:YAG lasers or with new tunable dye lasers, fluorescent measurements are now being extended out into the IR range where there is less possibility for interference with the emitted light. Fluorogenic dyes that emit light with wavelengths in the range from 0.7 to 1.5 μm are now being investigated. Since photomultiplier tubes are not as useful for wavelengths >1 μm, solid state detectors are more commonly used. The recording photodetector must have a wide dynamic response capable of quickly resolving huge differences in light intensity, on the order of a million times (six orders of magnitude) or more. Complications in interpreting fluorescent images include additional signals from natural autofluorescent biochemical processes, for example from NADH, that occur in plant and animal cells.

6.5.3 NADH Fluorescence

Chance (1991) has reviewed the scientific advances that have been made in measuring NADH fluorescence from biological systems where 340 nm excitation signals can generate NADH emission around 460 nm. Studies have been conducted to investigate differences between metabolic activation under aerobic and anaerobic conditions in isolated mitochondria, in isolated cells, and most recently, in intact tissues under *in vivo* conditions. Normal metabolic function could be maintained until O_2 fell below about 2%.

6.6 PHOSPHORESCENCE

When a phosphorescent material is illuminated with light, some light is absorbed, exciting it into a higher energy state. The energy must then be transferred either by light emission or some other process. This energy transfer is called quenching. Another chemical species may accelerate the quenching, although the time response could be limited by the diffusion rate of the quenching species. Practical applications of this property are possible when the lifetime τ of the phosphorescent material in the presence of a given concentration C of the quenching chemical species is long enough to be measured.

6.6.1 Basic Theory

The theory for the lifetime of the phosphorescent emission was described by Stern and Volmer (1919). The relationship is given by

$$\frac{\tau_0}{\tau} = 1 + k_q \tau_o C \tag{125}$$

where τ_0 is the lifetime in the absence of the quencher ($C = 0$), and the quenching parameter k_q is related to the combined rates of diffusional transport for the quenching agent and the phosphorescent material. Usually, the quenching agent is much more diffusible than the phosphorescent species. The relative light intensity is

$$\frac{I_0}{I} = 1 + (K_{eq} + k_q \tau_0) C + K_{eq} k_q \tau_0 C^2 \tag{126}$$

where I_0 is the phosphorescent light intensity in the absence of quencher, and K_{eq} is the association constant for binding of the quencher to the phosphorescent species. When $k_q \tau_0 \gg K_{eq}$, or if quenching is purely dynamic ($K_{eq} = 0$), then Equation (126) can be simplified to

$$\frac{I_0}{I} = \frac{\tau_0}{\tau} = 1 + k_q \tau_0 C \tag{127}$$

and both the lifetime and intensity are inversely related to the quencher concentration. The previous relationships have also been used to describe the decay of fluorescent emission when it is quenched by another chemical species.

If a biosensor membrane of thickness Δx and diffusivity D is controlling the transport of quenching agent, then

$$k_q = \frac{2D}{\Delta x^2} \tag{128}$$

can be substituted into Equations (125) and (126) as a first approximation for the diffusion-limited process. To have the optimum response time, the membrane should be freely permeable to the quenching agent and should be as thin as possible, as is also true for electrochemical sensors.

6.6.2 Deviation from Theory

It has been observed in many luminescent systems that I_0/I is not linearly related to the inverse lifetime [Equation (127)], and is often downward curved. This complicates the calibration of optical biosensors based on phosphorescence or fluorescence quenching. An empirical power law model

$$\frac{I_0}{I} = 1 + k_q \tau_0 C^n \tag{129}$$

has been used to correct for nonlinearity.

Recently, Carraway et al. (1991a) derived another mathematical model that is based on the relative contributions of static and dynamic quenching mechanisms in heterogeneous systems. The light intensity in their model is described by a series of Stern-Volmer relationships

$$\frac{I_0}{I} = \left[\sum_{i=1}^{n} \frac{f_{0i}}{1 + k_{qi} \tau_{0i} C} \right]^{-1} \tag{130}$$

with individual fractions

$$f_{0i} = \frac{I_{0i}}{\sum\limits_{i=1}^{n} I_{0i}} = \frac{\alpha_i \tau_i}{\sum\limits_{i=1}^{n} \alpha_i \tau_i} \tag{131}$$

where α_i are weighting constants. In order to compare lifetime and intensity measurements, they defined a weighted mean lifetime

$$\tau_M = \frac{\sum\limits_{i=1}^{n} \alpha_i \tau_i}{\sum\limits_{i=1}^{n} \alpha_i} \tag{132}$$

Also, a weighted mean lifetime in the absence of quencher τ_{M0} can be defined by substituting τ_{0i} for τ_i in Equation (132). Computer simulations were performed which confirmed the usefulness of the theoretical model for a wide range of heterogeneous systems.

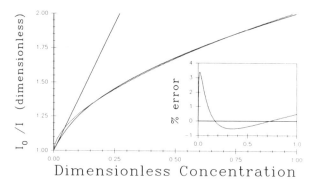

FIGURE 6.5. *Stern-Volmer linear (straight line) and nonlinear multicomponent [solid curve, Equation (130)] relationships between light intensity and quencher concentration. The best empirical model fit [dashed line, Equation (120)] to the nonlinear curve is also shown. Error for fit is shown in inset.*

The two nonlinear relationships for the light intensity with quencher concentration are shown in Figure 6.5 for the empirical Equation (129) (dashed line) and the multiple lifetime model [Equation (130)]. Values are calculated with three widely spaced relative values of $k_q\tau_{0i} = 10$, 1, and 0.1 and $f_{0i} = 1/3$ for each site (solid curve). The best fit of the empirical model to the multiple lifetime model is also shown for this example, with $n = 0.584$ and $k_q\tau_0 = 1.01$. If the linear Stern-Volmer relationship is used with an arithmetic mean $k_q\tau_0 = 3.7$ (straight line) for these three lifetimes to interpret the luminescent decay, it would clearly underestimate the true quencher concentration. The error for the best fit of the empirical relationship (shown in the inset of Figure 6.5) is fairly small, with the greatest deviation at low quencher concentrations. Although the empirical model may not be as accurate, it may be easier to fit to experimental data than the multiple lifetime model, and has been used by other investigators to correct for the nonlinearity.

6.6.3 Signal Measurement

Carraway et al. (1991b) used their model to interpret the photochemistry of an O_2 sensor using a luminescent transition-metal complex Ru(4,5-diphenyl-1, 10-phenanthroline)$_3^{2+}$ in silicon rubber. The Stern-Volmer plots for the data obtained with this sensor were found to be nonlinear. Static quenching was assessed to be a minor factor. By fitting both the intensity and lifetime data, they found that Equation (130) was better than the empirical Equation (129). Their data were consistent with a two-site model

[$n = 2$ in Equation (129)], with the second site much less reactive than the first.

6.7 OXYHEMOGLOBIN AND OXIMETRY

6.7.1 Basic Theory

Hemoglobin (Hb) is the specialized carrier protein that facilitates O_2 delivery from the lungs to the tissues. Each Hb molecule within the red blood cell is able to reversibly carry up to four O_2 molecules. There are also some dysfunctional hemoglobins that do not carry as much O_2, such as car-boxyhemoglobin (Hb combined with carbon monoxide), and methemoglobin. As the red blood cells travel through the microcirculation, they become progressively less oxygenated. The relative amount of O_2 bound to hemoglobin (HbO$_2$) is defined as the saturation (S), which can be expressed as either a fraction ($0 < S < 1$) or more commonly as a percent. There are a number of mathematical representations of the oxyhemogobin equilibrium curve. Probably the simplest is the Hill model

$$S = \frac{\left(\dfrac{P}{P_{50}}\right)^n}{1 + \left(\dfrac{P}{P_{50}}\right)^n} \tag{133}$$

where P_{50} is the O_2 partial pressure at 50% saturation and the exponent n is a pseudo-cooperativity factor. Around the midpoint, the model is fairly accurate, but not at the upper and lower ends. For human oxyhemoglobin, n is typically around 3 and P_{50} is around 27 Torr. Myoglobin, another protein carrier that facilitates O_2 transport, can be described by the Hill model with $n = 1$. This protein is especially found in heart and skeletal muscle tissues. In this special case, the mathematical model is similar to the single enzyme carrier model with P_{50} equivalent to K_m.

A more accurate, two-state (tense and relaxed) mathematical model by Monod et al. (1965) for the oxyhemoglobin equilibrium curve is represented by

$$S = \frac{LK_T P (1 + K_T P)^3 + K_R P (1 + K_R P)^3}{L (1 + K_T P)^4 + (1 + K_R P)^4} \tag{134}$$

where L is an allosteric constant, and the tense T and relaxed R state equilibrium constants are K_T and K_R respectively. There are several other theoretical and empirical models for the oxyhemoglobin equilibrium curve, and a significant number of published papers where the best parameters for individual models were obtained from human and animal blood saturation data.

6.7.2 Spectral Properties

The color shift from blue to red after blood has been oxygenated is a familiar property of blood. Light spectroscopy has been used successfully to quantify the degree of blood oxygenation. Light absorption changes with O_2 can be measured at specific wavelengths from transmitted light through uniform blood samples. The change in spectral properties for oxyhemoglobin is illustrated in Figure 6.6. Millikan (1942) was able to use these principles for hemoglobin oximetry, by placing yellow and green filters over each half of a photovoltaic cell. Later, Wood and Geraci (1949) determined the optimum wavelengths in the red ($\lambda = 640$ nm) and infrared ($\lambda = 805$ nm) regions, which permitted practical measurements. The light absorption in the infrared region does not change with oxygenation, and is referred to as an isobestic point, as shown in Figure 6.6.

The saturation can be calculated from the relative change in light absorption by

$$S = \frac{I_{\lambda=640}}{I_{\lambda=640} + I_{\lambda=805}} \times 100\% \qquad (135)$$

where I is the light intensity at the two wavelengths. Oximeters have also been developed to measure oxyhemoglobin saturation by comparing multi-

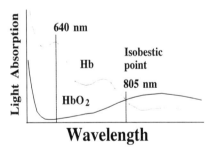

FIGURE 6.6. *Schematic drawing of light absorption as a function of light wavelength for oxygenated hemoglobin (lower curve) and deoxygenated hemoglobin (upper curve). Isobestic point where the curves intersect is used as a reference point for two wavelength oximeters.*

ple wavelengths. An eight-wavelength ear oximeter, described by Merrick and Hayes (1976), was produced commercially by Hewlett-Packard in 1970. Saturation was computed from the light transmitted (I_t) through human ear lobes at eight different wavelengths in the 650 to 1,050 nm range from

$$S = \frac{A_0 + \sum_{n=1}^{8} A_n \ln I_t}{B_0 + \sum_{n=1}^{8} B_n \ln I_t} \times 100\% \qquad (136)$$

where $A_0 - A_8$ and $B_0 - B_8$ are empirical constants. These constants were determined experimentally by taking arterial blood samples from human subjects as they breathed gases with different O_2 concentrations. However, these properties lump together scattering and absorption in the skin and blood of the ear lobe, and another set of constants would need to be determined for whole blood measurements. More recently, Schmitt (1991) has published a table listing absorption and scattering parameters for human blood at wavelengths of 660, 805, and 940 nm. Once the blood saturation is determined by oximetry, the blood PO_2 can be calculated from an algorithm for the oxyhemoglobin equilibrium curve.

6.7.3 Chemical Properties

Normal arterial blood with a hematocrit around 45% by volume is able to carry around 20 mL of O_2 per 100 mL of blood. This is nearly two orders of magnitude more O_2 than it is physically possible to carry dissolved in water or in blood plasma. Furthermore, the equilibrium kinetics for oxyhemoglobin binding are altered by temperature (T), pH, CO_2, and 2,3-diphosphoglycerate (DPG) in the blood, changing how readily O_2 can be released to tissue or picked up in the lung. Combined spectrophotometric and electrochemical measurements have been made in whole blood samples to characterize the chemical and spectral properties of the human oxyhemoglobin equilibrium curve.

Winslow and Rossi-Bernardi (1991) summarized some of the current theories for the cooperative binding of O_2 to hemoglobin and the role of the major allosteric factors (T, pH, CO_2, and DPG) on the equilibrium curve. The effects of the major allosteric factors have also been mathematically modeled by a number of different approaches. A blood algorithm has been developed by the author (Buerk and Bridges, 1986). A semi-empirical equilibrium model was fit to standard human blood data reported in the litera-

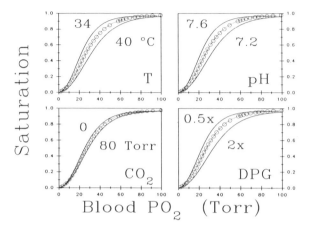

FIGURE 6.7. *Effect of temperature, pH, CO_2 and DPG on oxyhemoglobin equilibrium curve computed from an algorithm by Buerk and Bridges (1986). Data for human blood at standard conditions reported by Severinghaus (1966) is shown in each panel (open circles).*

ture and an algorithm was developed for computing nonstandard conditions, which is illustrated in Figure 6.7. The individual effects of each allosteric factor on human blood are shown in each panel, while holding the other three variables constant in the calculation. The model fit (dashed line) for the human oxyhemoglobin curve at standard conditions (pH = 7.40, T = 37°C, PCO_2 = 40 Torr and DPG/Hb = 0.9) from the data reported by Severinghaus (1966) (open circles) is shown in each panel, with corresponding deviations above and below it. At standard conditions, 50% of the maximum available O_2 is at a P_{50} of 26.9 Torr. Oxygen delivery to tissue is improved when the equilibrium curve is shifted to the right ($P_{50} > 26.9$), as occurs with increased T, more acidic conditions, increased PCO_2, or greater DPG. The clinical measurement of arterial blood PO_2 and the assessment of O_2 delivery to different organs of the body is a very important area, as discussed previously for electrochemical sensors. The medical instruments industry presently has over 40 manufacturers of oximetry and blood gas instruments.

6.7.4 Pulse Oximetry

Blackwell (1989) has reviewed the technological advances in oxyhemoglobin oximetry that have led to current clinical instruments for the noninvasive measurement of blood O_2 saturation and pulse rate. Microprocessors enable detection of pulsatile changes in the light signal, which are used to compute the heart rate. The microprocessor also allows corrections to be made for variations in the ambient light. However, pulse oximeters are not very accurate at lower blood saturations, where they do not follow the simple Lambert-Beer Law [Equation (113)]. The device is usually placed on the skin, and therefore depends on complex, heterogeneous optical properties and patterns of the blood flow through the microcirculation in the underlying tissues.

More elaborate modeling and data interpretation may be possible to improve these measurements. Schmitt (1991) published a table listing absorption and scattering parameters for human skin perfused with blood at wavelengths of 660, 805, and 940 nm. He also presented a more general theory for attenuation of light through various layers of the skin, based on different light absorption and scattering properties. Despite their lower accuracy, pulse oximeters have become especially useful as continuous clinical monitors to alert medical personnel to possible incidents of inadequate blood oxygenation.

6.7.5 Tissue Oximetry

Jöbsis (1977) was the first to report that near infrared light (wavelengths between 700 and 900 nm) could be used to transilluminate tissues to monitor not only oxyhemoglobin saturation, but the oxidation of the copper band of cytochrome c oxidase (cytochrome a,a_3) in the mitrochondria as well. Hampson and Piantadosi (1988) developed a laser-based near infrared spectroscopy instrument using a bank of GaAlAs laser diodes emitting light at 775, 810, 870, and 904 nm. The laser diodes were pulsed at 1 kHz with pulse durations of 200 nanoseconds. The intensity of the incident light was monitored with a photodiode and the transmitted light was measured with a photomultiplier tube. The complexity of the light absorption and scattering in the pathway has not allowed full deconvolution of the multiple wavelength spectra into units of concentration or absolute optical densities. An algorithm was developed to compute relative variations in optical density for oxyhemoglobin, total hemoglobin, and cytochrome a,a_3 from the detected light.

Because of the difficulty in interpreting optical spectra from living tissues, Ferrari et al. (1989) evaluated an alternate method where the first derivative of the spectrum was analyzed. A computer-controlled near infrared spectrometer using a rotating filter wheel was used to collect spectra in the range from 730 to 960 nm at a rate of 3 Hz. Measurements were made from the brains of eight anesthetized dogs using 5 mm diameter fiberoptic light bundles to transmit the incident light through the skull into the brain and to direct reflected light back to a silicon detector. The dogs were sub-jected to various hypoxic gas mixtures and sagittal sinus venous blood samples were taken for comparison with the optical data. The first deriva-tive of the spectra was found to enhance the changes due to oxyhemoglobin saturation and minimize changes due to differences in blood volume. An equation relating the first derivatives at two wavelengths, plus a term for the first derivative at a third wavelength, was used to calculate the blood saturation in brain tissue. A good correlation was found for the computed saturation and co-oximeter measurements of the sagittal sinus venous blood saturation. Undifferentiated spectra and second derivatives were also evalu-ated, with poor results. The first derivative method may be useful for mini-mizing the differences in wavelength-dependent absorption in different pa-tients where anatomical and geometrical relationships are highly variable.

6.8 DIGITAL IMAGE PROCESSING

Optical biosensors can benefit from advances in digital processing of the images or other types of signal processing techniques. Digital image pro-cessing is becoming increasingly common in new medical diagnostic tech-niques, such as computed radiology, tomography, magnetic resonance imaging, single-photon-emission computed tomography, and positron-emission tomography. These instruments use electromagnetic energy (X-rays, gamma rays, magnetic fields, etc.) outside the visible or IR light ranges. Enormous quantities of information are contained in the resulting images, which can be digitized according to the gray scale for each pixel. The factor limiting spatial resolution is the number of discrete detectors within the scanning device resulting in the increased cost of the instrument.

While many of these new medical diagnostic technologies are directed towards obtaining more detailed, three-dimensional structural images in-side the body, the internal biochemistry of cells and organs can also be studied. Fluorescence studies have been used to study the movement of in-tracellular ions, such as Ca^{++} using a dye like fura-2. There are many other luminescent reactions that can be followed now by optical methods, includ-ing fluorescent indicators for intracellular pH. Fiberoptic cables or optical waveguides can be coupled to detectors for use in different types of bio-sensors, as discussed in the following section.

6.9 OPTODES

In the early 1970s, Lübbers and Opitz (1976) coined the term "optodes" as a description for the various types of measurements that can be made with optical transducers, analogous to the use of electrodes for electrochemical transducers. Optically clear plastic fibers can transmit light with minimal losses over large distances, and can be made with relatively small dimensions. The use of single fibers or small bundles of fibers in optic cables has allowed miniaturization of quite a number of optical techniques in the past decade. Either a single optical channel, or a bifurcated channel—one to transmit light and the other to direct light back to a sensitive detector—can be used. Fiberoptic sensors for blood gas analysis, particularly for determining oxyhemoglobin saturation, have been the most successful commercial applications. Fiberoptic-based medical instruments do not have the safety problems that other technologies have, where electrical currents can be hazardous to patients and must be carefully controlled. The first fiberoptic biosensor was described by Schultz and Sims (1979). Although other types of fiberoptic biosensors have been developed since then, they have not yet achieved widespread use.

6.9.1 pH Optodes

An early design for a pH optode was developed by Peterson et al. (1980, 1984), who coupled a bifurcated fiberoptic cable to a small cavity containing a pH-sensitive dye. Through the Lambert-Beer Law, the pH can be related to the concentration C_{dye} of the dye and its buffering pK capacity by

$$\text{pH} = \text{p}K - \ln \left[\frac{\epsilon C_{dye} L}{\ln (I_0/I_m)} - 1 \right] \tag{137}$$

where I_0 is the incident light, I_m is the measured light, and ϵ is the extinction coefficient for a given light pathlength L. More recently, Besar et al. (1989) developed an LED-based fiberoptic system that can use either phenol red or BHD universal indicator. The respective measuring and reference wavelengths were 565 and 635 nm for phenol red and 635 and 930 nm for the universal dye. Ultrabright red or green LEDs were used for the reference light sources with a PIN photodiode used as the detector. It was possible to measure pH in the range from 5.5 to 8.5, with accuracies between 0.015 and 0.03 pH units with this optode.

6.9.2 Oxygen Optodes

Peterson et al. (1984) also developed a fiberoptic probe for O_2, based on the principle of fluorescence. A schematic of the probe is shown in Figure 6.8. Seventy different fluorescent dyes were considered, but the best characteristics were determined to be for the dye perylene dibutyrate (solvent

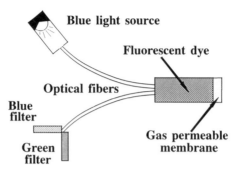

FIGURE 6.8. *Fiberoptic probe developed by Peterson et al. (1984) for measurement of O_2 by fluorescent quenching of a dye. The dye is excited by blue light and green light is emitted. The partial pressure of O_2 is determined from the ratio of light intensities.*

green 5). Another important factor for choosing this dye was that it is not toxic. The solvent green dye was encapsulated inside a rigid, gas-permeable tube of porous polypropylene with approximately 25 μm thick walls. The end was sealed after filling. Two 0.25 mm diameter optical fibers, either 90 or 120 cm long, had their ends terminating in the dye chamber. The final 30 cm of the fiberoptic pair leading into the chamber were threaded through a larger tube filled with carbon black to shield the optic fibers from ambient light. One fiber was used to transmit the excitation light from a 60 W deuterium (blue) light source and the other fiber picked up the fluorescent emission (green light) from the dye. The PO_2 could be related to the ratios of the blue and green light intensities (I) by

$$PO_2 = \text{gain} \cdot \left(\frac{I_{\text{blue}}}{I_{\text{green}}} - 1 \right)^m \tag{138}$$

where an exponent (m) was added to empirically correct the Stern-Volmer relationship [Equation (125)] for nonideal curvature. This is equivalent to the empirical model described previously [Equation (129)]. The step response to 98% completion was about two minutes. The sensitivity of the dye declined by about 3% per day during dry storage, but was much less (0.1% per day) when stored in water. Apparently something in the optical fiber itself was responsible for the desensitization of the dye. The probe was tested in animal blood (sheep) by inserting it through an 18 gauge catheter into the bloodstream of the carotid artery. The probe responded well for about 80 minutes. Clotting problems were encountered at that time. After cleaning the probe, the sensitivity was restored.

Wolthuis et al. (1992) describe an optode for O_2 based on a viologen compound in a 20% dipyridyl and 40% glycol film spin coated on glass. The viologen was excited by UV light, coupled through optical fibers. The absorption was monitored with a red LED and measured with a PIN photodiode. A particular advantage of this system is the possibility for sterilizing the transducer. Gamma radiation (2.5 mRad) sterilization was tested, causing only a 20% loss in sensitivity, nitrous oxide and halogenated anesthetic gases had no effect on the optode. This O_2 optode is envisioned as a disposable device, and preliminary tests indicated that it has a lifetime capable of over 250 measurements. It has not yet been tested *in vivo*.

Bernt and Lakowicz (1992) describe the use of a violet light (454 nm)–emitting solid state electroluminescent lamp (ELL) for an O_2 optode. This inexpensive light source can provide more power than blue LEDs, although aging effects were observed with these devices. Contrary to most previous methods, which are based on measuring light intensity, Bernt and Lakowicz measured the quenching lifetime of tris(4,7-diphenyl-1,10-phenylanthroline)ruthenium(II) chloride embedded in a silicon matrix. A PIN photodiode was used as the light detector. The phase shift induced by the fluorescence was measured, which depends on quenching lifetime and is independent of the light intensity. A 10 kHz square wave was used to drive the ELL and modulate the light intensity. In the absence of O_2, a 40° phase shift was seen. In room air, an 8° shift was measured. They concluded that the ELL device could be very useful, especially if a lamp output stabilization circuit is used to keep the light intensity constant as it ages. The ELL optode might be able to measure O_2 quenching decay times as short as 30 nanoseconds.

Surgi (1989) reviewed some of the indicator molecules that have been used for fiberoptic-based O_2 optodes. These include perylene dibutyrate, decacyclene, pyrene, 5-(4-bromo-1-naphthoyl)pentyl-trimethylammonium bromide, *N*-methylacridone, and Pt(II) or Ru(II) derivatives of α-diimine ligands. He described tests for O_2 optodes based on *N*-methylacridone-coated silica on Teflon membranes. The indicator was excited at 400 nm and fluorescence emission monitored at 460 nm. The fluorescence quenching lifetime was found to have short (about 6.5 nanoseconds) and long (about 50 μseconds) components, with the longer component more suitable for practical measurements of quenching lifetimes. The 90% response time of the optode was about 12 seconds when switching from N_2 to O_2, but was longer (about 42 seconds) when the opposite change was made.

6.9.3 PCO$_2$ Optodes

Kawabata et al. (1989) described a PCO_2 sensor using fluorescein dye as a pH indicator, based on the same principle as discussed previously in Chapter 3. A single fiber design with the tip ground at an angle was used. A xenon arc lamp with wavelength adjusted to 490 nm was used as the excitation signal and a photomultiplier tube was used as the detector, with a mechanical light chopper modulating the light signals at 80 Hz. The fluorescein was immobilized on the fiberoptic tip in a mixture of high and low weight poly(ethylene glycol) at 5×10^{-7} mol/g. The pH of the polymer was adjusted to 7, and the total thickness of the dried polymer was about 10 μm. A particular advantage of this design was the lack of an aqueous buffer, which could evaporate and alter the optode sensitivity.

6.9.4 Enzyme Modified Optodes

Luo and Walt (1989) have described a general method for directly attaching enzymes to the surface of single optical fibers for enzyme-based optodes. The active end was first polished to a smooth finish, then cleaned in concentrated sulfuric acid for several hours and rinsed in distilled water. The fiber was silanized by soaking in a solution of 10% γ-(methacryloxy) propyltrimethoxysilane in toluene for 24 hours. After washing and drying, the silanized tip was immersed in a mixture of 1 mL N,N-methylenebis-(acrylamide) and 2 mL N-(3-aminopropyl)methacrylamide hydrochloride in which 100 μL of ammonium persulfate was added. These reagents were dissolved in a phosphate buffer with pH $= 7.0$. This mixture was allowed to polymerize, then the optical fiber was removed. The polymerized tip was then allowed to soak for three hours in a 1 mL solution containing 5 mg of the vitamin sulfosuccinimidyl 6-(biotinamido)hexanoate in 0.05 M sodium bicarbonate at pH 8.5 to 9. The biotin-vitamin-coated tip was then transferred to a phosphate buffer solution containing 3 to 5 mg of avidin (from egg white) for 24 hours under refrigeration.

This procedure produced a stable avidin/biotin film on the optical fiber, which was then used to covalently immobilize different enzymes labeled with the pH-sensitive dye (fluorescein). The resulting fluorescence intensity was monitored following excitation with a xenon arc lamp. Good results were obtained with a penicillin optrode using immobilized penicillinase [EC 3.5.2.6, type I from *Bacillus cereus*] and with an ethyl butyrate optrode using immobilized esterase [EC 3.1.1.1]. A urea optrode using immobilized urease was not as stable.

6.10 OPTICAL WAVEGUIDES

The principle for optical waveguides, shown schematically in Figure 6.9, is similar to optical fibers, except that a planar conductor of light is used. A

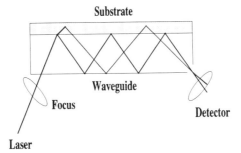

FIGURE 6.9. *Principle of optical waveguide measurement. Laser light transmitted through the waveguide can penetrate into the surface substrate and excite the photoactive species. The resulting emitted light can be detected from the phase shift of interfering light coming out of the waveguide.*

glass substrate can be coated with a thin dielectric film, 0.1 to 10 μm in thickness, which has a lower refractive index. A bioactive substrate is placed over this surface. Most of the light transmitted into the device has multiple reflections as it travels through the medium. However, some of the light can penetrate up into the substrate. This light is reflected back into the waveguide with a shift in phase that can interfere with the transmitted light. Changes in properties within the substrate layer can be followed by detecting the changes in interference. The light source can also be used to excite fluorescent material in the substrate layer, and to examine the change in the light spectrum coming out of the device.

6.10.1 Multiple Attenuated Total Reflection

Mendelson et al. (1990) used an 8 W (maximum) tunable CO_2 laser for multiple attenuated total reflection measurements by Fourier transform spectroscopy in the near infrared range to determine glucose concentrations in human and pig blood. The spectral resolution was within the range from 10^{-6} to 10^{-3} cm^{-1}. The wavelength at 9.676 μm was monitored where peak glucose absorption occurs. The spectrum from distilled water was also measured, and subtracted from the blood spectrum to enhance the glucose component. An advantage of this technique is that the light penetration into the blood was only about 1.3 μm, so the physical size of the blood sample was not important. When transmitted light is used, it is necessary to have very small chambers with thin blood layers. Also, heat absorption from the light source was not a problem with such a small penetration depth. A nonzero, constant offset absorption was found, indicating interference from other molecules (probably proteins). There was a good correlation for the optically measured changes in absorption when compared to blood glucose measurements made with a commercially available electrochemical glucose biosensor (Model 23A, Yellow Springs Instruments).

6.11 LIGHT-ADDRESSABLE POTENTIOMETRIC SENSOR

Parce et al. (1989) designed and tested a device for microphysiological measurements. It uses a silicon semiconductor sensor, which is activated when it is illuminated with light to measure the electrical potential on its surface. Optic fibers direct light to small, localized regions of the sensor. The site of the measurement can be varied by illuminating different regions of the device with a light-emitting diode (LED). The sensor surface is fabricated by first growing a 30 nm thick SiO_2 film, then coating a 100 nm thick layer of Si_3N_4 by low-pressure chemical vapor deposition. Finally, the surface is coated with an optically transparent conductive layer of indium-tin oxide. The light-addressable potentiometer sensor (LAPS) measures the pH of the medium within the device, from a voltage transient that is measured after it is activated by the LED. A measurement around 1 μV/minute is equivalent to about 0.001 pH unit/minute.

Prior to applying indium-tin oxide, an additional 1 μm thick layer of SiO_2 is deposited by steam oxidation. A photolithographic pattern is created and an array of cavities is formed by anisotropic etching in SF_6-C_2ClF_5 gas plasma. After the final indium-tin oxide coating, an array of wells with active surfaces on the walls and cavity floors is created on the sensor, with inactive spaces in between due to the unetched, thick SiO_2 layer. Each well is approximately 50×50 μm square and 50 μm deep, with 25 μm thick walls. The cavity wall angle is very steep, typically $>85°$ from the horizontal. Molecular Devices Corporation (Menlo Park, CA) has released a commercial version of the LAPS-based microphysiometer (Cytosensor™ microphysiometer). Growth factor responses, interactions between cytokines and lymphokines, receptor and signal transduction methods, and responses to antagonists and agonists have been studied with this device by a number of laboratories. As described further in Chapter 9, the LAPS device can also be loaded with living cells for additional types of physiological testing.

6.12 REFERENCES

Arnold, M. A. 1991. "Fluorophore- and Chromophore-Based Fiberoptic Biosensors," in *Biosensor Principles and Applications*, L. J. Blum and P. R. Coulet, eds., New York, NY: M. Dekker, Inc., pp. 195–211.

Berndt, K. W. and J. R. Lakowicz. 1992. "Electroluminescent Lamp-Based Phase Fluorometer and Oxygen Sensor," *Anal. Biochem.*, 201:319–325.

Besar, S. S. A., S. W. Kelly and P. A. Greenhalgh. 1989. "Simple Fibre Optic Spectrophotometric Cell for pH Determination," *J. Biomed. Eng.*, 11:151–156.

Blackwell, G. R. 1989. "The Technology of Pulse Oximetry," *Biomed. Instrum. Technol.*, pp. 188–193.

Blum, L. J. and S. M. Gautier. 1991. "Bioluminescence- and Chemiluminescence-Based Fiberoptic Sensors," in *Biosensor Principles and Applications*, L. J. Blum and P. R. Coulet, eds., New York, NY: M. Dekker, Inc., pp. 213–247.

Buerk, D. G. and E. W. Bridges. 1986. "A Simplified Algorithm for Computing the Variation in Oxyhemoglobin Saturation with pH, PCO_2, T and DPG," *Chem. Eng. Commun.*, 47:113–124.

Carraway, E. R., J. N. Demas and B. A. DeGraff. 1991a. "Luminescence Quenching Mechanisms for Microheterogeneous Systems," *Anal. Chem.*, 63:322–336.

Carraway, E. R., J. N. Demas, B. A. DeGraff and J. R. Bacon. 1991b. "Photophysics and Photochemistry of Oxygen Sensors Based on Luminescent Transition-Metal Complexes," *Anal. Chem.*, 63:337–342.

Chance, B. 1991. "Optical Method," *Annu. Rev. Biophys. Biophys. Chem.*, 20:1–28.

Ferrari, M., D. A. Wilson, D. F. Hanley, J. F. Hartmann and R. J. Traystman. 1989. "Determination of Cerebral Venous Hemoglobin Saturation by Derivative near Infrared Spectroscopy," in *Oxygen Transport to Tissue – IX*, K. Rakusan, G. P. Biro, T. K. Goldstick and Z. Turek, eds., New York, NY: Plenum Press; *Adv. Exp. Med. & Biol.*, 248:47–53.

Hampson, N. B. and C. A. Piantadosi. 1988. "Near Infrared Monitoring of Human Skeletal Muscle Oxygenation during Forearm Ischemia," *J. Appl. Physiol.*, 64:2449–2457.

Jöbsis, F. F. 1977. "Noninvasive, Infrared Monitoring of Cerebral and Myocardial and Circulatory Parameters," *Science*, 198:1624–1627.

Kawabata, Y., T. Kamichika, T. Imasaka and N. Ishibashi. 1989. "Fiber-Optic Sensor for Carbon Dioxide with a pH Indicator Dispersed in a Poly(ethylene glycol) Membrane," *Anal. Chim. Acta*, 219:223–229.

Lou, S. and D. R. Walt. 1989. "Avidin-Biotin Coupling as a General Method for Preparing Enzyme-Based Fiber-Optic Sensors," *Anal. Chem.*, 61:1069–1072.

Lübbers, D. W. and N. Opitz. 1976. "Quantitative Fluorescence Photometry with Biological Fluids and Gases," in *Oxygen Transport to Tissue – II*, J. Grote, D. Reneau and G. Thews, eds., New York, NY: Plenum Press; *Adv. Exp. Med. & Biol.*, 75:65–68.

Mendelson, Y., A. C. Clermont, R. A. Peura and B-C. Lin. 1990. "Blood Glucose Measurement by Multiple Attenuated Total Reflection and Infrared Absorption Spectroscopy," *IEEE Trans. Biomed. Eng.*, 37:458–465.

Mendelson, Y. 1991. "Invasive and Noninvasive Blood Gas Monitoring," in *Bioinstrumentation and Biosensors*, D. L. Wise, ed., New York, NY: M. Dekker, Inc., pp. 249–279.

Merrick, E. B. and T. J. Hayes, 1976. "Continuous, Non-Invasive Measurements of Arterial Blood Oxygen Levels," *Hewlett-Packard J.*, 28:2–9.

Millikan, G. A. 1942. "The Oximeter," *Rev. Sci. Instrum.*, 13:434–444.

Monod, J., J. Wyman and J. Changeaux. 1965. "On the Nature of Allosteric Transitions: A Plausible Model," *J. Mol. Biol.*, 12:88–118.

Parce, J. W., J. C. Owicki, K. M. Kercso, G. B. Sigal, H. G. Wada, V. C. Muir, L. J. Bousse, K. L. Ross, B. R. Sikic and H. M. McConnell. 1989. "Detection of Cell-Affecting Agents with a Silicon Biosensor," *Science Wash. DC*, 246:243–247.

Peterson, J. I., S. R. Goldstein, R. V. Fitzgerald and D. K. Buckhold. 1980. "Fiberoptic pH Probe for Physiological Use," *Anal. Chem.*, 52:864–869.

Peterson, J. I. and G. Vurek. 1984. "Fiber-Optic Sensors for Biomedical Applications," *Science*, 123:123–127.

Peterson, J. I., R. V. Fitzgerald and D. K. Buckhold. 1984. "Fiberoptic Probe for *in vivo* Measurement of Oxygen Partial Pressure," *Anal. Chem.*, 56:62–67.

Schmitt, J. M. 1991. "Simple Photon Diffusion Analysis of the Effects of Multiple Scattering on Pulse Oximetry," *IEEE Trans. Biomed. Eng.*, 38:1194–1203.

Schultz, J. S. and G. Sims. 1979. "Affinity Sensors for Individual Metabolites," *Biotechnol. Bioeng. Symp.*, 9:65.

Severinghaus, J. W. 1966. "Blood Gas Calculator," *J. Appl. Physiol.*, 21:1108–1116.

Stern, O. and M. Volmer. 1919. "Über Die Abklingungszeit der Fluoreszenz," *Physik. Z.*, 20:183.

Surgi, M. R. 1989. "Design and Evaluation of a Reversible Fiber Optic Sensor for Determination of Oxygen," in *Applied Biosensors*, D. L. Wise, ed., Boston, MA: Butterworths, pp. 249–290.

West, S. J., S. Ozawa, K. Seiler, S. S. S. Tan and W. Simon. 1992. "Selective Ionophore-Based Optical Sensors for Ammonia Measurement in Air," *Anal. Chem.*, 64:533–540.

Winslow, R. M. and L. Rossi-Bernardi. 1991. "Oxygen-Hemoglobin Dissociation Curve," in *The Lung: Scientific Foundations*, R. G. Crystal, J. B. Wester, P. J. Barnes, N. S. Cherniak and E. R. Weibel, eds., New York, NY: Raven Press, Ltd., pp. 1225–1231.

Wolthuis, R. S., D. McRae, J. C. Hartl, E. Saaski, G. L. Mitchell, K. Carcin and R. Willard. 1992. "Development of a Medical Fiberoptic Oxygen Sensor Based on Optical Absorption Change," *IEEE Trans. Biomed. Eng.*, 39:185–193.

Wood, E. H. and J. E. Geraci. 1949. "Photoelectric Determination of Arterial Oxygen Saturation in Man," *J. Lab. Clin. Med.*, 34:387–401.

CHAPTER 7

Miscellaneous Transducer Technologies

7.1 ENZYME-BASED CALORIMETRY

All of the biochemical reactions discussed in the previous chapters involve a change in molar enthalpy (ΔH). For example, the reaction with glucose catalyzed by glucose oxidase [Chapter 4, Equation (91)] releases 80 kJ/mol. The change in temperature due to chemical reactions that take place for the different biosensor designs discussed so far has been assumed to be negligible. Isothermal conditions are generally assumed when interpreting the biosensor signal. Either the thermal mass of the biosensor is so large that heat is rapidly dissipated, or the temperature of the entire measuring device is regulated with a circulating water bath or an electrically heated metal block.

Calorimeters have been used in chemistry for a long time. Modern calorimeters are automated and highly sensitive instruments. Their principle of operation is based on heat generated (exothermic reaction) or absorbed (endothermic reaction) from the environment after completing the chemical reaction in a closed system. Besides determining the heat of vaporization for pure compounds and the molar enthalpies for simple chemical reactions, there are other applications for calorimeters, including determination of liquid-phase heat capacities and their temperature dependence, and determining vapor-liquid equilibrium for multicomponent systems.

7.1.1 Theory

The total amount of heat (Q) produced or gained within the calorimeter can be related to the change in temperature (ΔT) from

$$Q = -n_p \Delta H = C_s \Delta T \qquad (139)$$

where n_p is the total moles of product and C_s is the overall heat capacity of the system where the reaction takes place. By thermally insulating the reaction chamber (adiabatic conditions), the heat losses or gains by conduction to or from the environment can be minimized, and ΔT caused by the reaction can be accurately measured. Of course, this is a nonspecific measurement, and calorimeters cannot discriminate between different chemical reactions. If multiple reactions occur, only the net temperature change from the combined heat change as a result of all of the enthalpy changes for the individual reactions can be measured.

7.1.2 Transducers

There are many types of temperature transducers that could be used in calorimeters. Thermistors are probably the most convenient, and very small thermistor beads, around 0.1 mm in diameter, are available. Thermistors are ceramic semiconductors made from sintered mixtures of metal oxides which have an electrical resistance (R) that decreases with temperature in a very nonlinear fashion, described empirically by

$$\frac{1}{T} = a + b \ln R + c(\ln R)^2 \tag{140}$$

where T is in Kelvin and a, b, and c are constants. The resistance at room temperature is in the kΩ range, with temperature coefficients typically -3 to -6% per $^\circ$C for the more commonly used thermistors. The resistance change with temperature can be readily measured in a Wheatstone bridge circuit with sensitivities of 100 mV per 0.001 $^\circ$C. Unlike electrochemical sensors, there is essentially no drift in the physical properties of thermistors with time, although there can be drift in the electronic instrumentation. Temperature measurements can be made repeatedly and rapidly with great accuracy.

Another method for quantifying heat production would be to monitor the power delivered to a feedback-regulated electrical heater that is maintaining a biosensor at a constant temperature. When extra heat is produced by a chemical reaction, less power is needed. Alternately, if the reaction is endothermic, more power would be required to maintain the temperature.

Microcalorimeters can be calibrated by injecting known volumes and concentrations of chemical species that either generate or absorb a precise amount of heat from mixing. The change in energy can be measured for enzyme-mediated chemical reactions in simple solutions, or can be used to measure changes in energy production of living cell cultures in response to flow-injected substrates. It is also possible to have a differential calorimeter design, where the chemical reaction of interest does not occur in one of the channels.

7.1.3 Applications

Flow through calorimeter systems have been developed based on the measurement of temperature changes in the outflow stream or within the reaction chamber. This type of analysis is usually based on a pulse injection of the analyte, which is then carried into the reactor where the specific enzymes are immobilized. The temperature and flow rate of the input stream must be well regulated to make accurate measurements. Also, there can be no gas bubbles introduced during injection or formed within the reactor. The transient change in temperature can be analyzed from the peak of the curve, by integrating the area under the curve, or by more sophisticated mathematical modeling and curve fit optimization techniques.

Danielsson (1991) reviewed research conducted at the University of Lund in Sweden on enzyme-based flow through calorimeters. A glucose biosensor was designed based on the calorimeter principle, immobilizing both glucose oxidase and catalase. The catalase reaction

$$\text{catalase}$$
$$2H_2O_2 \rightarrow O_2 + 2H_2O \tag{141}$$

generates 100 kJ per mole of H_2O_2, which more than doubles the total enthalpy change for a given concentration of glucose. A similar design was also used for a lactate biosensor immobilizing lactate oxidase and catalase. Lactate oxidase catalyzes the following reaction

$$\text{lactate oxidase}$$
$$\text{L-lactate} + O_2 \rightarrow \text{pyruvate} + H_2O_2 \tag{142}$$

and the catalase reaction creates more heat as H_2O_2 is consumed. Coenzyme recycling techniques, discussed previously in Chapter 4, have also been useful for increasing the heat of reaction and allowing detection of much lower concentrations of analyte. Danielsson (1991) reported much greater sensitivity with a biosensor that coimmobilized lactic oxidase with lactate dehydrogenase. When NADH is present, the latter enzyme catalyzes the reaction

$$\text{lactate dehydrogenase}$$
$$\text{pyruvate} + \text{NADH} + H^+ \rightarrow \text{L-lactate} + \text{NAD}^+ \tag{143}$$

allowing lactate to reenter the primary reaction [first step in Equation (141)] and produce more heat. Amplification factors of around 1,000 were obtained, and lactate concentrations as low as 10 nM could be detected.

Danielsson (1991) reported that a miniaturized calorimeter instrument with 0.1 to 0.2 diameter channels using very low flow rates of 25 to 50 μL/min for injected sample volumes of 1 to 10 μL had been constructed and was undergoing further evaluation. Bäckman and Wadsö (1991) from the University of Lund constructed a small (3.3 mL) calorimetric vessel, shown schematically in Figure 7.1, which can be used either as a batch reactor or as a flow through reactor. A miniature Clark O_2 electrode and pH electrode were also inserted into the chamber, which was stirred at 100 r.p.m. by a rotating turbine blade. The shaft of the stirrer was hollow, so that fluid could flow through the shaft into the chamber. The temperature changes measured for different experimental conditions were corrected for the energy imparted by the stirrer. The correction factor was a function of the flow rate through the system, and was determined from experimental measurements.

7.2 PIEZOELECTRIC MICROBALANCES

Piezoelectric transducers can be used to detect very small changes in mass (piezoelectric microbalance) that occur on their surfaces, as shown schematically in Figure 7.2. Usually synthetic quartz crystals, which are cut at either 35°15′ (AT-cut) or 49°00′ (BT-cut) relative to the plane of the crystal structure, are used for the piezoelectric element. Gold, aluminum, nickel, or other metals are vapor deposited on opposite sides of the crystal to allow electrical connections. The crystal is then inserted into a feedback loop of a broadband radio frequency amplifier.

7.2.1 Theory

The potential field generated in the feedback circuit causes a mechanical vibration to occur. Oscillations occur at resonant frequencies in the range from 5 to 15 MHz for most commercially available crystals. The vibration frequency becomes slower as mass accumulates on the crystal surface. When the crystal is in air, the shift in frequency is approximately linear with changes in mass (Δm), as given by the Sauerbrey (1959) relationship

$$\Delta f = \frac{2f_0^2 \Delta m}{A\sqrt{\varrho\sigma}} \tag{144}$$

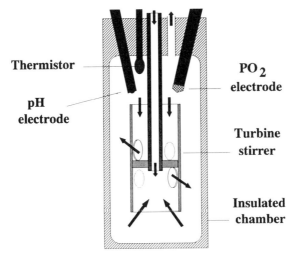

FIGURE 7.1. *Microcalorimetric vessel with sample volume of 3.3 mL designed by Bäckman and Wadsö (1991) at the University of Lund in Sweden. Heat production rate is measured with thermistor (±0.3 μW), with conventional electrodes for pH (±0.01 unit) and O_2 (±4 μM/L). The vessel can be used either in the batch mode (closed) or as a flow through reactor using cultured cells or microbes. Sample is stirred with turbine blade.*

where A is the surface area, f_0 is the resonant frequency, ϱ is the density, and σ is the shear modulus for the quartz crystal. This relationship assumes that the surface mass is also rigid, which may not always be true.

When the transducer is in contact with liquid, the resonant frequency is altered by the physical properties of the liquid. Kanazawa and Gordon

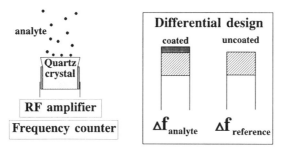

FIGURE 7.2. *Principle for piezoelectric measurement of mass on surface of a quartz crystal microbalance (left) and operation in differential mode (right). The uncoated crystals tend to oscillate at a fundamental resonant frequency which can be accurately measured by a frequency counter. The frequency of oscillation will slow down as biomaterial (circles) is adsorbed on the surface, increasing the mass of the transducer.*

(1985) propose that the resonant frequency $f_{o,L}$ in liquid relative to the value in air f_0 is given by

$$f_{o,L} = f_0 \left(1 - \sqrt{\frac{f_0}{\pi} \frac{\varrho_L \mu_L}{\varrho_Q \sigma_Q}} \right) \tag{145}$$

where ϱ is the density, μ is the viscosity of the liquid, σ is the elastic shear modulus for the quartz crystal, and the subscripts L and Q refer to liquid and crystal respectively. Very high sensitivities can be achieved in either dry or wet modes of operation, with theoretical detection limits on the order of 10^{-11} to 10^{-10} g when the frequency counter has 0.1 Hz accuracy. For example, the sensitivity of a piezoelectric microbalance sensor with area of 0.35 cm^2 described by Ebersole et al. (1991) was 3.2×10^{-9} g for each 1 Hz change in frequency.

Piezoelectric crystals will not oscillate in very dense or viscous fluids. Also, piezoelectric transducers immersed in liquids become more temperature-sensitive due to the relatively greater changes in the liquid properties with temperature compared to the temperature-dependent changes in the crystal alone. Equation (145) may not be adequate for some operational conditions, and more elaborate modeling may be required to fully characterize the behavior of piezoelectric microbalances exposed to liquids. Duncan-Hewitt and Thompson (1992) have recently presented a four-layer theory, incorporating the possibility that there is fluid slip at the interface, causing incomplete coupling of energy. The four layers are: solid sensor, liquid adjacent to the surface, a transition zone, and the bulk liquid far from the sensor. Besides calculating the shift in resonant frequency, the model also can be used to predict the impedance and shift in phase angle for different fluid and sensor properties.

7.2.2 Applications

Various detection schemes are possible with piezoelectric transducers, as recently reviewed by Luong and Guilbault (1991). The surface of the piezoelectric microbalance can be coated with a biologically active film that can influence the adsorption process and rate of mass accumulation, or be designed such that only specific biochemical substrates will be attracted and adsorbed. Both the attached film and the substrate layer that is absorbed on the transducer surface must remain stable as the crystal vibrates.

It is very difficult to model and predict effects of different polymers and films on the frequency response characteristics of modified transducers. A trial and error approach has often been necessary, as perhaps exemplified by the piezoelectric CO_2 gas sensor developed by Fatibello-Filho et al. (1989) for a possible application in fermentation monitoring. They reported test results for 20 different coatings, most of which had poor stability or poor reproducibility. Some materials were found to be totally insensitive to CO_2. The best material for their application was tetrakis(hydroxyethyl)-ethylenediamine. The material was dissolved in acetone, and the piezoelectric electrodes were coated and baked to form a film. The optimum mass of coating was also determined by trial and error. The final design produced a 430 Hz change in frequency for 10% (v/v) CO_2 under test conditions where the temperature was 25°C and the gas flow rate was 100 mL/min. The device was tested for temperature sensitivity and for potential interfering chemical species expected in fermentation processes, including ethanol, acetic acid, acetaldehyde, 1-butyric acid, propionic acid, acetoin, methanol, and acetone. Trace gases including SO_2, H_2S, CS_2, CH_3-SH, CH_4, and NH_3 were also tested.

Water, ethanol, acetaldehyde, and acetone caused the most interference. Water vapor was removed for most of the tests by running the gas samples through a column containing 50 g of molecular sieve. This was effective for input humidities up to 70%. Other methods to remove interfering factors were also tested, including hydrophobic membranes and desiccants. Although about 15% of the CO_2 was absorbed by the molecular sieve, the CO_2 detector was still sensitive for gas flow rates between 60 and 230 mL/min. CO_2 absorption affected the measurements at low $CO_2 < 1.8\%$. The calibration was linear over the range from 1.8 to 16% CO_2. At higher CO_2, the device became saturated.

Some of the early applications of the piezoelectric microbalance were as immunosensors, which will be discussed further in Chapter 8. There are a number of commercial instruments that use piezoelectric microbalance technology for detecting changes in dust, smoke, or specific chemicals in air, using various surface modification techniques.

7.3 SURFACE ACOUSTIC WAVE TRANSDUCERS

These devices also use the piezoelectric phenomenon, except that the electrodes are usually formed on the same side of the crystals rather than on opposite sides. The contact electrodes are usually formed as an interdigitated pattern, as illustrated in Figure 7.3. As one electrode induces the piezoelectric vibration, a Rayleigh surface acoustic wave is created which travels to the other electrode, where a delay in the propagated wave can be detected. The resonant frequency f_0 for surface acoustic wave transducers can be much higher than piezoelectric microbalances, and devices operating in the GHz range have been designed.

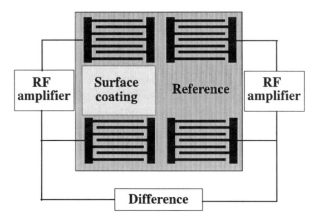

FIGURE 7.3. *Differential configuration for an interdigitated surface acoustic wave transducer with chemical selectivity determined by type of surface coating.*

7.3.1 Theory

Ballantine and Wohltjen (1989) have reviewed the physical principles of surface acoustic wave devices. The frequency change seen by an electrode pair with an isotropic, nonconducting film of thickness h with density ϱ and shear modulus σ coated between them is given by

$$\Delta f = f_0^2 h \left[(k_1 + k_2)\varrho - k_2 \frac{4\sigma}{V_R^2} \frac{\lambda + \sigma}{\lambda + 2\sigma} \right] \tag{146}$$

where k_1 and k_2 are constants for the piezoelectric material, V_R is the Rayleigh wave velocity and λ is the Lamb constant. The first term is similar to Equation (144) and is related to the mass of the film layer, while the second term represents the elastic properties of the film. If the film is very elastic, the second term may be negligibly small. Other waveforms can be generated, which would require a different analysis. As with the piezoelectric microbalance, the interactions between the transducer and fluid interfaces become much more complicated to model.

7.3.2 Applications

So far, the majority of practical applications for surface acoustic wave transducers have been for detecting chemical vapors. As we have seen for other transducer types, it is convenient to have a differential measurement. The configuration illustrated in Figure 7.3 is a dual surface acoustic wave delay line, with a different frequency shift depending on the propagated wave path across the surface coating (left side) or across the uncoated piezoelectric element (right side). Alternately, designs with two different surface coatings can be made. The difference between the two fundamental frequencies on the two sides can be monitored. As material is adsorbed on the specialized coating, the frequency difference will increase. The differential configuration also minimizes fluctuations in temperature or pressure, since both transducers are exposed to the same conditions.

Ballatine and Wohltjen (1989) reviewed some of the chemical vapor transducers using this technology. Styrene and vinyl acetate with detection limits of 5 ppm have been measured on $PtCl_2$(ethylene)(pyridine) films and cyclopentadiene has been measured on poly(ethylene maleate) films. Gases including H_2 NH_3, NO_2, H_2S, and SO_2 can be measured. Humidity sensors have also been designed based on the surface wave acoustic principle.

7.4 CHEMOMECHANICAL HYDROGELS

A number of polymers change their physical properties, reversibly swelling or shrinking as their water content varies with the substrate pH, ionic concentration, or temperature. Enzymes can be immobilized within these hydrogels. For example, Kost et al. (1985) describe a glucose-sensitive hydrogel, made by immobilizing glucose oxidase. In the presence of glucose, gluconolactone is formed [Equation (91)] and spontaneously decomposes to gluconic acid. As a result, the pH of the gel changes. More acidic conditions cause the water content to increase and the gel to swell. This alters the electrical properties of the hydrogel, which can be measured by conventional conductimetric sensors under the gel membrane. Alternate techniques could be developed to exploit these hydrogel properties. For example, a chemomechanical biosensor may be possible if the gels exert sufficient force on a strain gauge, piezoelectric element, or other mechanical transducer. McCurley and Seitz (1991) exploited this concept with an optical transducer. The swelling of sulfonated polystyrene (Dowex 50W) and sulfonated dextran (SP Sephadex) polymers with different strengths of ionic solutions were quantified. This was accomplished by measuring the change in refractive index of light reflected off of a flexible surface that was physically displaced as the polymers were swelling.

Osada et al. (1922) have recently described a synthetic gel that is capable of movement with electrical stimulation. The gel is a weakly cross-linked poly(2-acrylamido-2 methyl propane) sulfonic acid. A strip of gel 1 mm $\times$ 5 mm $\times$ 20 mm was immersed in a 20 mM pyridium chloride, 30 mM sodium sulfate solution. This lead to an expansion in the volume of the

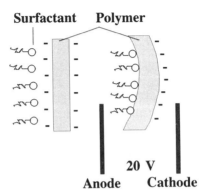

FIGURE 7.4. *Schematic drawing of a mechanical change due to osmotic induced polymer swelling in response to electrical stimulation.*

gel by 45 times. As shown schematically in Figure 7.4, the block of gel can reversibly change shape after applying a DC potential. As current flows through the gel, one side of the polymer shrinks, while the other swells. A strip of gel was made with two hooks at either end and placed on a racheted guide to allow only unidirectional movement. A 20 V DC potential was applied through carbon electrodes, alternating polarity every 2 seconds. A maximum velocity of 25 cm/min was achieved with this synthetic gel. It may be possible to make much smaller gel fibers for physically propelling miniaturized devices by this technology.

7.5 LIQUID CRYSTAL SENSORS

Liquid crystals change their optical properties with temperature and other factors. Zhu and Hieftje (1990) exploited the fluorescent properties of the liquid crystal N,N'-bis(p-butoxybenzylidene)-α,α'-bi-p-toluidine. A thin layer of liquid crystals was applied to both sides of a thin glass microscope slide cover. The liquid crystals were excited by a continuous wave argon-ion laser at a wavelength of 351.1 nm. A fluorescent emission spectrum was measured with a peak around 539 nm at room temperature. This device was placed into a flowing stream of heated air at 200°C. The fluorescent spectrum peak was shifted to 607 nm at this temperature. The liquid crystal transducer was used to detect anthracene vapor. This is a polynuclear aromatic hydrocarbon that has carcinogenic and mutagenic properties. The liquid crystal transducer could detect anthracene vapor at concentrations as low as 6.8×10^{-10} M/cm^3 of gas. The transducer was reversible, and had a response time of around 2 min.

7.6 ENZYME REACTORS WITH HIGH PERFORMANCE LIQUID CHROMATOGRAPHY

The concept of using enzymes or other biological elements to convert an analyte into another chemical species that is more readily detected by a transducer is also useful for gas chromatography. The effluent from flow injection systems using immobilized enzymes can be directed to a high performance liquid chromatography (HPLC) instrument to detect the products of the reaction. Yao (1989) reviewed some of the research conducted in this area. Some of the earlier attempts involved mixing soluble enzymes with the effluent from a reactor, but this method can be very expensive for some enzymes. It is more economical to have an immobilized enzyme reactor. However, the flow rate and dispersion of the chemical species traveling through a reactor affect the efficiency of the conversion reaction, which may not be at its optimum rate.

7.6.1 Applications

Yao (1989) described two flow through enzyme reactor systems coupled to HPLC as well as to electrochemical transducers. A system for detecting acetylcholine and choline using acetylcholinesterase and choline oxidase was tested. A small stainless steel column (inside diameter 0.2 mm, length 20 mm) was packed with LiChrosorb NH_2 (Merck) with 10 μm particle size on which the enzymes were immobilized. The immobilized enzymes retained 95% of their activity after three months. The efficiency of the reactor with varying flow rate was tested in the range from 0.5 to 4 mL/minute. The flow had little effect on the conversion of acetylcholine to choline, but the choline reaction efficiency decreased with increasing flow, reaching a plateau about 15 to 20% below the maximum efficiency obtained at the slowest flow rate. This was not a serious problem, since the choline reaction was still quite efficient. The lower limits of detection for choline and acetylcholine were 1.2 and 1.8 $\times$ 10^{-12} M respectively. Another system for detecting purine bases was also described by Yao (1989). The HPLC column was slightly larger (inner diameter 4 mm, length 12 mm). The enzymes purine nucleoside phosphorylase, guanase and xanthine oxidase were co-immobilized onto the LiChrosorb NH_2 particles. Reactions were similar to the last three steps of Equation (100) described previously for the fish freshness biosensor. Different purine derivatives were injected into the system. Purine bases including purine, xanthine, hypoxanthine, guanine and adenine could be detected. Also the nucleosides xanthosine, inosine, guanosine and adenosine could be detected. The purine nucleotides (ATP, ADP, AMP, GTP, GMP, etc.) and purine alkaloids (caffeine, theophylline) did not have any effect on the measurements.

Commercial HPLC systems are available that also have conventional electrochemical transducers included in the flow stream. Sometimes an additional advantage of the flow through reactor design is the physical separation of the analyte from other, potentially interfering chemical species. For example, in the choline detection system described above, Yao (1989) reported that ascorbic acid preceded and dopamine lagged behind the choline signal. Thus biosensors or electrochemical transducers in the flow stream may be free from these interferences if the separation is great enough. High performance liquid chromatography technology is likely to achieve wider applications and could easily be modified by including specific types of biosensors.

7.7 REFERENCES

Bäckman, P. and I. Wadsö. 1991. "Cell Growth Experiments Using a Microcalorimetric Vessel Equipped with Oxygen and pH Electrodes," *J. Biochem. Biophys. Meth.*, 23:283–293.

Ballantine, D. S., Jr. and H. Wohltjen. 1989. "Surface Acoustic Wave Devices for Chemical Analysis," *Anal. Chem.*, 704A–713A.

Danielsson, B. 1991. "Enzyme Thermistor Devices," in *Biosensor Principles and Applications*, L. J. Blum and P. R. Coulet, eds., New York, NY: M. Dekker, Inc., pp. 83–106.

Duncan-Hewitt, W. C. and M. Thompson. 1992. "Four-Layer Theory for the Acoustic Shear Wave Sensor in Liquids Incorporating Interfacial Slip and Liquid Structure," *Anal. Chem.*, 64:94–105.

Ebersole, R. C., R. P. Foss and M. D. Ward. 1991. "Piezoelectric Cell Growth Sensor," *Bio/Technol.*, 9:450–454.

Fatibello-Filho, O., J. F. de Andrade, A. A. Suleiman and G. G. Guilbault. 1989. "Piezoelectric Crystal Monitor for Carbon Dioxide in Fermentation Processes," *Anal. Chem.*, 61:746–748.

Kanazawa, K. K. and J. G. Gordon. 1985. "The Oscillation Frequency of a Quartz Resonator in Contact with a Liquid," *Anal. Chim. Acta*, 175:99–105.

Kost, J., T. A. Horbett, B. D. Ratner and M. Singh. 1985. "Glucose-Sensitive Membranes Containing Glucose Oxidase: Activity, Swelling, and Permeability Studies," *J. Biomed. Mat. Res.*, 19:1117–1133.

Luong, J. H. T. and G. G. Guilbault. 1991. "Analytical Applications of Piezoelectric Crystal Biosensors," in *Biosensor Principles and Applications*, L. J. Blum and P. R. Coulet, eds., New York, NY: M. Dekker, Inc., pp. 107–138.

McCurley, M. F. and W. R. Seitz. 1991. "Fiber-Optic Sensor for Salt Concentration Based on Polymer Swelling Coupled to Optical Displacement," *Anal. Chim. Acta*, 249:373–380.

Osada, Y., H. Okuzaki and H. Hori. 1992. "A Polymer with Electrically Driven Motility," *Nature*, 355:242–244.

Sauerbrey, G. 1959. "Verwendung von Schwingquarzen zur Wagung dunner Schichten und zur Mikrowagung," *Z. Phys.*, 155:206–222.

Yao, T. 1989. "Bioelectroanalytical Flow Systems with Immobilized Enzymes," in *Applied Biosensors*, D. L. Wise, ed., Boston, MA: Butterworths, pp. 321–348.

Zhu, C. and G. M. Hieftje. 1990. "Feasibility of Using Liquid Crystals for the Development of Molecularly Selective Fiber-Optic Chemical Sensors," *Anal. Chem.*, 62:2079–2083.

CHAPTER 8

Immunosensors

The human immune system is extraordinarily complex, and antigen-antibody interactions are not fully understood at the present time. Antibodies are Y-shaped protein molecules which are composed of equal numbers of heavy and light polypeptide amino acid chains held together with disulfide bonds. These highly specialized proteins are able to recognize and bind only certain types of antigen molecules at receptor sites on the tips of each arm. Many mammalian antibodies are in the immuno-gamma-globulin (IgG) class, with molecular weights around 160,000 daltons. Biotechnological advances in cloning and culturing hybrid cells have permitted the production of monoclonal and polyclonal antibodies that are specific to a chosen antigen or a group of closely related chemical species. Some of these antibodies can be manufactured in relatively large quantities without great expense by exposing cultured cells or microbes to an antigen. It may also be possible to manipulate antibody production using site-directed mutagenesis to create new, synthetic antibodies with antigen specificities that are not normally possible. Therefore, there may be an infinite number of possible immunosensors using antibodies that only detect certain antigens.

There are many practical applications for immunosensors if they can be reliably made. Immunosensors may be useful for quantifying how well the human immune system is functioning, and could serve as valuable clinical diagnostic tools. There may also be significant applications in identifying environmental contaminants. Although there has been a great deal of scientific research on immunosensors, starting in the early 1970s, commercial immunosensors are just beginning to emerge into the marketplace.

Immunosensors can be divided into two general categories: nonlabeled types that rely on some change in physical properties, and labeled im-

163

munoassays that rely on the direct detection of a specific label. Schematic drawings for the interactions between antibody and antigen, and competitive reactions with additional antibodies are shown in Figure 8.1. Immunosensors can be developed by incorporating either the antigen or the antibody on the sensor surface, although the latter design is used most often. Since the immunocomplex reactions that occur with antigens and antibodies are highly specific, extremely precise sensitivities at the molecular level are possible. However, it is still possible to have nonspecific interactions, as illustrated in Figure 8.1. These interactions, which can include adsorption of proteins, changes in fluid viscosity and density, or other physical changes near the surface, may be important for some types of transducers and less important for others. Another problem is that some immunoreactions are not reversible, so that only a single immunoassay is possible. Considerable research efforts have been directed towards the development of renewable antibody surfaces or for maintaining reagent concentrations so that repetitive immunoassays can be made without loss of sensitivity.

8.1 POTENTIOMETRIC IMMUNOSENSORS

There are several types of potentiometric immunosensors. The principle of operation common to each type is a measurable change in electrical potential that occurs when the combined surface charges are altered after an

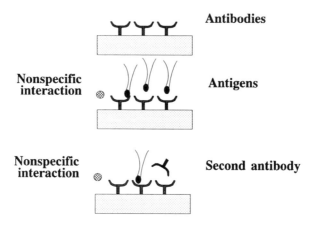

FIGURE 8.1. *Principle of immunosensor sensitivity. An antibody is immobilized on the surface of the sensor (top panel) which is highly specific for a given antigen (middle panel). Further exposure of the immunosensor to other antibodies can be made to achieve precise molecular recognitions.*

immunocomplex forms. All three types are classified therefore as non-labeled sensors.

8.1.1 Modification of Electrode

The first type of immunosensor involves modification of the electrode surface by covalently bonding either the antigen or the antibody. The change in electrode potential after immunocomplex formation is then measured directly by the electrode. The magnitude of the change depends on the ionic composition of the surrounding medium.

8.1.2 Modification of Membrane

The second type of immunosensor uses an electrode covered by a modified membrane, with either antigen or the antibody bound on its surface, or contained within the membrane itself. The change in transmembrane potential is measured by the electrode after an immunocomplex forms on the outer membrane of the sensor. Again, ionic compositions in the fluids on both sides of the membrane play a role in the measured potential change.

8.1.3 Modification of Solid State Device

The third type of immunosensor determines the surface potential on the gate of a field effect transistor that has been covered with an antibody binding membrane. The resulting change in the electrical field modulates the resistance of the gate, as discussed previously (Chapter 5).

8.1.4 Catalytic Antibodies

Another immunosensor design employs catalytic antibodies that cause selective catalysis which generates acid products, leading to an acidic change in pH. The pH change is measured potentiometrically. For example, Blackburn et al. (1990) described a biosensor for phenyl acetate and similar compounds using the catalytic antibody 20-G-9. A 3 μL drop of solution containing the antibody was allowed to soak into a membrane, which was then placed directly over a 2.5 mm diameter pH electrode with a flat surface. The outer surface was covered with a dialysis membrane. Since the combined membranes were relatively thick, the response was slow. Logarithmic calibrations with sensitivities in the range from 13 to 22 mV/log concentration were found, depending on the external buffer. The sensitivity was found to be higher in 0.1 mM compared to 1 mM Tris-HCl buffer. The lower detection limit for phenyl acetate was 5 μM. The biosensor had an excellent lifetime, with some biosensors still sensitive after being stored wet for one year.

8.2 AMPEROMETRIC IMMUNOSENSORS

Other electrochemical techniques including amperometric detection schemes have been investigated for immunosensors. For example, Xu et al. (1990) describe a flow injection technique with dual glassy carbon working electrodes for the amperometric detection of 4-aminophenol in maternal serum. An immunoassay procedure was developed using mouse anti-human IgG for alpha-fetoprotein and compared with a commercial kit. Oxidation peaks were obtained in the flow injection system at flow rates of 1 mL/min using a 20 μL sample loop. Alpha-fetoprotein is a normal developmental glycoprotein and tests for its presence are useful for detecting birth defects. For example, in Down's syndrome its concentration is abnormally low. With spina bifida and open neural tube birth defects, its concentration is abnormally high. The flow injection immunoassay was found to be more sensitive than the commercial kit.

8.2.1 Capacitance Measurements

Another electrochemical method, where capacitance changes are measured in response to a sinusoidal voltage, was investigated for use in an immunosensor by Billard et al. (1991). They attached antibodies to the top surface of a silicon semiconductor treated with different silanes. The bottom side of the semiconductor was vapor deposited with a layer of gold to provide an electrical connection. In this application, the top of the semiconductor surface must remain electrically insulated from the external fluid sample. Cyanosilane proved to be ineffective for this purpose. Capacitance changes could be measured on surfaces treated with δ-aminobutyldimethyl-methoxysilane, using 0.1% glutaraldehyde to cross-link the antibodies. With a 14 mV amplitude, 10 Hz sinusoidal signal, they were able to measure a 400 pF/cm² change in capacitance with 10 μg/mL of toxin. However, the accuracy of their device was limited to 40 pF, so the lower limit of detection was only 1 μg/mL of toxin.

8.3 ENZYME-LINKED IMMUNOASSAYS

If a chemical substrate involved in an immune reaction can be converted into another chemical species by an enzyme-catalyzed reaction, immunosensors can be developed using the electrochemical principles as described previously for other enzyme-based sensors in Chapter 4. Several types of enzyme-linked immunosensors have been described by Aizawa (1991). For example, the antibody anti-α-fetoprotein (AFP) was bound to a membrane covering a Clark-type O_2 electrode. The immunosensor was immersed in solutions containing different amounts of catalase-labeled AFP. This caused differing amounts of catalase-labeled AFP to become attached to the membrane. After thorough washing, the immunosensor was placed in a reaction chamber with a fixed volume of buffer solution. O_2 electrode responses were measured after injecting a known amount of H_2O_2 into the reaction chamber. The catalase label converted the H_2O_2 to O_2, causing an increase in the O_2 electrode reading above the baseline level of dissolved O_2 initially present in the system. The responses were rapid, reaching steady state within 30 seconds. A calibration curve was made for AFP in the range of 5×10^{-11} to 5×10^{-8} g/mL, and a standard deviation of 15% was found for 25 repeated measurements at 5×10^{-9} g/mL AFP. The calibration curve was not linear for this immunosensor, and in fact, the O_2 electrode current increase was greatest at the lowest concentrations of AFP.

Another enzyme-linked sensor was described by Aizawa (1991) for the detection of the deadly poison ochratoxin A (OTA) which some bacteria can synthesize. The biosensor was again based on the conversion of H_2O_2 to O_2 by catalase. A catalase-labeled antibody specific to OTA was also used, but in this case, the toxin was directly bound to the sensor membrane and the antibody was present in the test solution. Tests were conducted with three different concentrations of the labeled antibody. OTA concentrations as low as 1×10^{-11} g/mL could be detected.

8.3.1 Redox-Mediated Immunosensor

As with enzyme-based biosensors, electron transfer in immune reactions can also be accomplished with redox mediators. This modification may allow current amplification for some types of immunosensors. Umaña et al. (1988) applied this principle to an immunosensor for the antigen phenytoin (5,5-diphenylhydantoin) using glucose oxidase with a polypyrrole-ferrocene redox mediator. As diagrammed in Figure 8.2 for generalized immunoreaction, their immunosensor was based on blocked electron exchange through the mediator. A ferrocene-phenytoin conjugate was synthesized, and a polyclonal anti-phenytoin antibody prepared. A glassy carbon electrode was modified with glucose oxidase and pyrrole-ferrocene. Two experimental conditions were tested. In the presence of glucose oxidase with excess glucose (>20 mM), the current depended on the catalytic

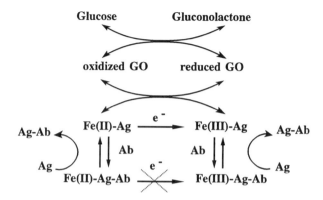

FIGURE 8.2. *Use of redox mediator for electron transfer in an immunosensor design by Umaña et al. (1988). The immunocomplex inhibits electron transfer through the ferrocene ion.*

rate of ferrocene with glucose oxidase, and was independent of scan rate. The overall current was given by

$$I = nFAC_0\sqrt{DkC_{enzyme}} \qquad (147)$$

where n is the number of electrons, A is the electrode area, k is the rate constant, C_{enzyme} is the glucose oxidase concentration, C_0 is the initial concentration, and D is the diffusivity of the electroactive species. In the absence of glucose oxidase, the limiting current was found to be a function of the scan rate ν, given by

$$I_{med} = \text{constant} \cdot AC_0\sqrt{n^3D\nu} \qquad (148)$$

with the constant around 2.69×10^5 for their system.

8.4 PIEZOELECTRIC MICROBALANCE IMMUNOSENSORS

As discussed previously in Chapter 6, the frequency shift of the quartz microbalance can be used to detect mass changes as material binds to its surface. This principle was first employed for a piezoelectric microbalance immunosensor by Shons et al. (1972), who coated a crystal with plastic, then immobilized bovine serum albumin on the surface. A frequency shift was measured after exposing the sensor to bovine serum albumin antibodies. The immunosensor required only a few minutes to make a measurement. This was much faster than a conventional passive agglutination method, which required hours to complete. Furthermore, the immunosensor was found to be just as accurate as the older method. However, there are still some uncertainties involved in the piezoelectric microbalance measurement technique. The primary source of error can come from nonspecific binding of proteins or other biomaterials into the activated surface. The other error can come from changes in the fluid viscosity, as discussed previously (Chapter 7). Another problem is the loss of the material coating the surface after washing and renewal of antibodies.

Luong et al. (1990) evaluated several techniques for attaching anti-*Salmonella typhimurium* antibodies to the surface of an AT cut piezoelectric crystal with a fundamental frequency of 9 MHz. The worst method was treatment with γ-aminopropyltriethoxysilane in benzene, which caused only an 80 Hz change in frequency when exposed to 10^9 *Salmonella typhimurium* cells/mL. The best method was the direct cross-linking of the antibody to the crystal treated with bovine serum albumin and 2.5% glutaraldehyde. After attaching the antibodies, the immunosensor was washed, then dipped in a phosphate solution with 0.1 M glycine to block unreacted aldehyde groups. The immunosensor had a 530 Hz frequency change with 10^9 cells/mL. Immunosensors made with the antibody immobilized on a biotin-avidin coating, or with the antibody immobilized on a polyethyleneimine polymer layer had intermediate sensitivities. The immunosensor was able to detect a lower limit of 10^5 cells/mL when incubated for five hours, and 10^7 if incubated for only 30 minutes. The immunosensor could be reused by washing with 8 M urea, but had a large drop in sensitivity after about six surface renewals. The sensitivity of the immunosensor to *E. coli* was minimal, with 10^9 cells/mL causing only a 40 Hz change in frequency.

8.4.1 Differential Design

In an attempt to circumvent the problems caused by nonspecific interactions, Roederer and Bastiaans (1983) designed a differential immunosensor by coating two piezoelectric crystals with glycidoxypropyltrimethoxysilane (GOPS). One crystal was used as a reference, the other was coated with the goat antibody to IgG. The differential immunosensor was tested in antigen solutions, and the resulting shift in frequency was found to be linear for antigen in the concentration range from 0.0225 to 2.25 mg/mL. The lower limit of detection was 13 μg/mL. The immunosensor surface could be renewed by washing with high ionic strength solutions. However, the sensitivity was not sufficiently high for practical applications. More recently, Davis and Leary (1989) designed a piezoelectric immunosensor that had a much greater sensitivity, with a frequency change of 1 Hz per 10 ng of mass.

A compensating circuit was used to improve the efficiency of the crystal oscillator. The liquid exposed surface was coated with protein A and tested in solutions containing rabbit or human IgG. Reproducible decreases in the frequency were measured. The addition of sheep anti-human IgG further decreased the frequency by a factor of three. The surface of the immunosensor was easily renewed by washing in an acidic buffer at pH = 3, without removing the protein A coating.

8.5 OPTICAL IMMUNOSENSORS

A number of different fiberoptic or other optical waveguides have been developed for immunosensors. A general type of bifurcated optic fiber design is illustrated in Figure 8.3 with two commonly used tip configurations. Single fiber designs have also been used. The light source is delivered to the tip and the transmitted or reflected light is picked up by a light detector. Arnold (1991) has reviewed some of the principles for both enzyme- and antibody-based measurements with fiberoptics, and the many chemical modifications for attaching the enzymes or antibodies to the surfaces on which the reactions take place. In the right panel of Figure 8.3(a), the antibodies are suspended in a microcavity behind a dialysis membrane permeable to the antigen. Optical changes that occur in the microcavity can be monitored. Other designs bind the antibody or antigen to the membrane surface where direct contact is made with the sample, as shown in the left

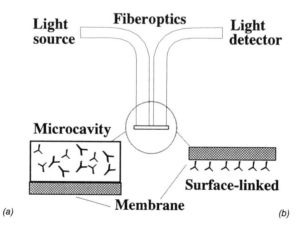

FIGURE 8.3. Two types of immunosensor tips for bifurcated fiberoptic design. (a) Antibodies are unbound, in fluid-filled microcavity separated from sample by a membrane. (b) Antibodies are bound on surface of membrane in direct contact with sample.

panel of Figure 8.3(b). Various optical techniques have been investigated for detecting changes in optical properties that result from the interaction of antibody and antigen on the surface. The measurements can be complicated by scattering and nonspecific absorption processes.

8.5.1 Light Scattering

Sutherland et al. (1984a) were able to measure changes in light intensity due to light scattering effects on a glass slide coated with antibodies. The slide was illuminated with light at a wavelength around 440 nm. In essence, the glass slide was acting as a light waveguide, with the immunoreaction on the surface causing the measured changes in light scattering.

8.5.2 Light Absorbance

Sutherland et al. (1984b) used a quartz optical waveguide with antibody covalently attached to the surface to study antibody binding of methotrexate. Light was transmitted through the waveguide at a wavelength of 310 nm, and was estimated to penetrate approximately 90 nm into the surface coating. With increased methotrexate binding, light was absorbed at a wavelength around 300 nm, primarily due to a benzoyl group in the molecule. The change in absorbance was related to methotrexate concentration, with a lower detection limit of 0.26 μM.

8.6 BIOLUMINESCENT IMMUNOASSAY

There have been research efforts to develop conjugates of antibodies or antigens with enzymes such as luciferase, which would emit light during a reaction. Jablonski (1985) covalently cross-linked a bacterial luciferase from *V. harveyi* with either *Staphylococcus aureus* protein A, or with anti-human IgG. Both conjugates retained their light-emitting ability. This bioluminescent immunoassay was compared with a radioimmunoassay method used commercially for detecting human rubella immunity, with favorable results. Aizawa (1991) has also discussed other electrochemiluminescent labels, such as luminol. Immunocomplex formations with antibodies can interfere with the electrically stimulated luminescent response.

8.7 FLUORESCENCE IMMUNOASSAY

There are numerous fluorescent probes that can be used to label antibodies or antigens. The fluorescence during immunoreaction can then be measured as the labels are replaced. The fluorescence can be detected by direct imaging through a microscope, through optical fibers, or through optical waveguides.

8.7.1 Optical Fibers

Vo-Dinh et al. (1991) describe a fiberoptic system for measuring DNA from human placental samples. A monoclonal antibody from mouse spleen cells was used to detect benzo[a]pyrene tetrol after mild acid hydrolysis of human placental tissue samples. The tip design of their immunosensor was similar to the microcavity design shown previously in Figure 8.3(a). A 10 mW He-Cd laser at 325 nm was used with emission detected by a photomultiplier tube through a 40 nm bandpass filter centered at 400 nm.

8.7.2 Controlled Release System

Barnard and Walt (1991) developed a competitive fluoroimmunoassay with a fiberoptic sensor using the controlled release of labeled antibodies to maintain sensitivity, which is shown schematically in the left panel of Figure 8.4. An antibody was labeled with fluorescein and an immunoglobulin G was labeled with Texas Red. When the antibody and IgG form an immunocomplex, the two fluorophor labels are very close to one another, allowing nonradiative transfer of energy. When the fluorescein molecule is excited by light, it donates energy to the Texas Red fluorophor, enhancing its fluorescent light emission. Fluorescein was excited at 480 nm and peak

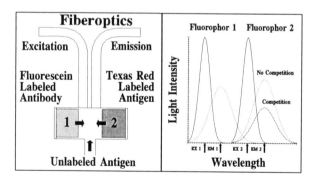

FIGURE 8.4. *Competitive fluoroimmunoassay with sustained release of reagents designed by Barnard and Walt (1991). Labeled antibody and antigen are released from polymer reservoirs and fluorescence measured by fiberoptics (right panel). The fluorescence emission from the second fluorophor (Texas Red) is reduced when unlabeled antigen competes with the reaction (left panel).*

emission monitored at 520 nm. Texas Red was excited at 570 nm with peak emission monitored at 610 nm.

A competitive reaction scheme was devised, where the analyte was unlabeled IgG. Two controlled release polymer reservoirs were fabricated using ethylene vinyl acetate, which continually released fluorescein-labeled antibody (reservoir 1) and Texas Red–labeled IgG (reservoir 2) into a reaction chamber. After an initial hydration period of approximately two days, the release rates from both reservoirs were constant and the immunosensors remained sensitive for 30 days. Longer lifetimes may be possible with greater loading or larger polymer reservoirs. Barnard and Walt (1991) tested sensors with only a single concentration (500 μg/mL) of unlabeled IgG, cycling with solutions with no IgG present. The analyte entered the reaction chamber through an opening, which could have variable dimensions to optimize the diffusion time required. When the unlabeled IgG concentration in the reaction chamber was high, it competed with the labeled IgG. Less energy was transferred to the Texas Red fluorophor, causing a decrease in its fluorescence emission, as shown schematically in Figure 8.4 (right panel). The concentration of unlabeled IgG could be calculated from the ratios of excitation and emission wavelengths for each fluorophor, with a correction factor for the excitation of Texas Red by the lower wavelength light used for the excitation of fluorescein. Because of the large physical dimensions of the reservoirs, reaction chamber, and analyte pathway, the response time was very slow. However, this device can be used for continuous monitoring over a relatively long time period, whereas other devices that require renewal of immunoreaction surfaces can only provide discontinuous measurements.

8.7.3 Liposome Amplification

Recently, Choquette et al. (1992) used planar waveguide technology to measure antibody-antigen fluorescence, using liposomes to augment the antigen concentration entering immunoreaction. A small flow channel (20 mm $\times$ 1.2 mm $\times$ 0.4 mm) with total volume of 9.2 μL was constructed on the glass surface of a planar waveguide coated with a thin layer of dielectric film to reflect light. The waveguide was tested with an He-Ne laser (632.8 nm wavelength) and was found to have modest optical losses, around 20%. An immunosensor for theophylline was tested, using an antibody prepared from mouse anti-theophylline IgG attached to the waveguide surface with 3-glycidoxypropyltrimethoxysilane. In order to increase the concentration of antigen reaching the antibodies, they prepared antigen-tagged liposomes, incorporating theophylline-conjugated phosphatidylethanolamine into the lipid membrane. Fluorescence experiments were conducted with an argon-ion laser excitation source, using the 488 nm wavelength to quantify changes in fluorescent emission, with corrections for background scattering. The laser power was reduced to minimize photobleaching losses. Theophylline standards in the range from 2×10^{-10} to 2×10^{-5} M were tested. Nonspecific adsorption was also tested with γ-globulin. Antigen-tagged liposomes were introduced by the flow injection technique, then the flow was stopped to allow equilibrium. For the lowest concentrations, up to 1 hour was required to reach equilibrium. Antibody activity was regenerated by exposing the liposomes to the detergent 1-O-octyl-β-D-gluco-pyranoside to disrupt the membranes, followed by a thorough washout. There was a significant loss in sensitivity with repeated measurements at the lower concentrations, down by approximately 50% after 12 samples. However, the sensitivity at the upper concentration ranges was not affected as much. The immunosensor sensitivity to theophylline in the clinically important range from 10 to 20 mg/L was fairly stable.

8.8 SURFACE RESONANCE

An optical technology, illustrated in Figure 8.5, called biospecific interaction analysis (BIA) has been developed to study the binding properties of biomolecules. An optical biosensor system based on this technology is commercially available (BIAcore™, Pharmacia Biosensor AB, Piscataway, NJ). The principle of detection is based on surface plasmon resonance, a phenomenon where energy is transferred from incoming photons to electrons on a metal surface. The reflected light for a specific wavelength will cancel at a certain incident angle (the "non-reflectance" angle). The change

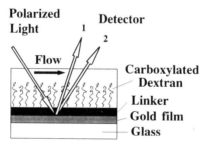

FIGURE 8.5. *Principle of operation for a flow through surface resonance immunosensor. A highly reflective gold surface is activated with a ligand linker, then covered with a layer of carboxylated Dextran. Polarized light is reflected off the surface and the shift in the region of minimum light intensity is measured as different antibodies and antigens are injected.*

in optical properties occurs at the flow channel surface when biomolecules are bound to a specific protein ligand (linker) coated on a thin gold film. The linker is then covered with a covalently bound carboxylated dextran layer, which provides an immobilizing matrix and eliminates nonspecific binding by direct adsorption. Polarized light illuminates the sensor surface, which has a total detection area of approximately 0.2 mm². The shift in the nonreflectance angle (from 1 to 2 in Figure 8.5) is detected as the optical properties change with binding. Similarly, the changes in optical properties with dissociation can also be measured. The immunosensor output is expressed in resonance units (RU), defined as 1,000 RU = 0.1° shift in the nonreflectance angle. These changes can be directly related to changes in mass concentration in the medium near the immunosensor flow channel surface.

The BIAcore™ system is modularly designed with four parallel flow channels on removable sample chambers. Each flow cell is 2.1 × 0.55 × 0.05 mm for a total volume of 60 nL. Sample volumes from 1 to 50 μL can be used. A fluid sample containing the bioactive material is delivered to the detecting area, which has been designed as an integrated unit on a removable module. The automated delivery of fluids and sensing is controlled by computer. A particular advantage of this system is that the surface of each immunosensor can be renewed for 50 to 100 cycles (depending on the stability of the linking ligand) by washing with hydrochloric acid. Typical analysis times require only 5 to 10 minutes, and reproducibilities are reported to be >95%. The time course of change can be followed, allowing estimation of kinetic parameters for binding or dissociation.

8.9 LASER MAGNET IMMUNOASSAY

Japanese researchers at Nippon Telegraph and Telephone Corporation have developed a new measurement technology consisting of a magnetic field generator and focusing system, using a laser to detect optical changes in the sample. A suspension of AIDS virus was magnetically labeled using ultrafine magnetic particles. The virus can then be concentrated at a local region by focusing the magnetic field. Known amounts of purified antigen to the virus were diluted with human blood serum, and the sensitivity of the laser measurement system was tested. The optical changes produced by the magnetic field were measured for several concentrations of antigen. The detection sensitivity was found to be 1×10^{-13} g/mL, at least 100 times more sensitive than other reported methods.

It is hoped that a more sensitive measurement of the antigen would lead to earlier detection of AIDS, since the production of antibodies may not occur for three months to one year after infection. This might assist in starting earlier treatment schedules.

8.10 REFERENCES

Aizawa, M. 1991. "Immunosensors," in *Biosensor Principles and Applications*, L. J. Blum and P. R. Coulet, eds., New York, NY: M. Dekker, Inc., pp. 249–266.

Arnold, M. A. 1991. "Fluorophore- and Chromophore-Based Fiberoptic Biosensors," in *Biosensor Principles and Applications*, L. J. Blum and P. R. Coulet, eds., New York, NY: M. Dekker, Inc., pp. 195–211.

Bäckman, P. and I. Wadsö. 1991. "Cell Growth Experiments Using a Microcalorimetric Vessel Equipped with Oxygen and pH Electrodes," *J. Biochem. Biophys. Meth.*, 23:283–293.

Barnard, S. M. and D. R. Walt. 1991. "Chemical Sensors Based on Controlled Release Polymer Systems," *Science Wash. DC*, 251:927–929.

Billard, V., C. Martelet, P. Binder and J. Therasse. 1991. "Toxin Detection Using Capacitance Measurements on Immunospecies Grafted onto a Semiconductor Substrate," *Anal. Chim. Acta*, 249:367–372.

Blackburn, G. F., D. B. Talley, P. M. Booth, C. N. Durfor, M. T. Martin, A. D. Napper and A. R. Rees. 1990. "Potentiometric Biosensor Employing Catalytic Antibodies as the Molecular Recognition Element," *Anal. Chem.*, 62:2211–2215.

Choquette, S. J., L. Locascio-Brown and R. A. Durst. 1992. "Planar Waveguide Immunosensor with Fluorescent Liposome Amplification," *Anal. Chem.*, 64:55–60.

Davis, K. A. and T. R. Leary. 1989. "Continuous Liquid-Phase Piezoelectric Biosensor for Kinetic Immunoassays," *Anal. Chem.*, 61:1227–1230.

Jablonski, E. 1985. "The Preparation of Bacterial Luciferase Conjugates for Immunoassay and Application to Rubella Antibody Detection," *Anal. Biochem.*, 148:199–206.

Luong, J. H. T., E. Prusak-Sochaczewski and G. G. Guilbault. 1990. "Development of a Piezoimmunosensor for the Detection of *Salmonella typhimurium*," in *Enzyme Engineering 10*, H. Okada, A. Tanaka and H. W. Blanch, eds., *Annals N.Y. Acad. Sci.*, 613:439–443.

Roederer, J. E. and G. J. Bastiaans. 1983. "Microgravimetric Immunoassay with Piezoelectric Crystals," *Anal. Chem.*, 55:2333–2336.

Shons, A., F. Dorman and J. Najarian. 1972. "An Immunospecific Microbalance," *J. Biomed. Mater. Res.*, 6:565–570.

Sutherland, R. M., C. Dahne and J. Place. 1984a. "Preliminary Results Obtained with a No-Label, Homogeneous Immunoassay for Human Immunoglobulin G," *Anal. Lett.*, 17:43–55.

Sutherland, R. M., C. Dahne, J. F. Place and A. S. Ringrose. 1984b. "Optical Detection of Antibody-Antigen Reactions at a Glass-Liquid Interface," *Clin. Chem.*, 30:1533–1538.

Umaña, M., J. Waller, M. Wani, C. Whisnant and E. Cook. 1988. "Enzyme-Enhanced Electrochemical Immunoassay for Phenytoin," *J. Res. Natl. Inst. Stand. Technol.*, 93:659–661.

Vo-Dinh, T., J. P. Alarie, R. W. Johnson, M. J. Sepaniak and R. M. Santella. 1991. "Evaluation of the Fiber-Optic Antibody-Based Fluoroimmunosensor for DNA Adducts in Human Placenta Samples," *Clin. Chem.*, 37:532–535.

Xu, Y., B. Halsall and W. R. Heineman. 1990. "Heterogeneous Enzyme Immunoassay of Alpha-Fetoprotein in Material Serum by Flow-Injection Amperometric Detection of 4-Aminophenol," *Clin. Chem.*, 36:1941–1944.

CHAPTER 9

"Living" Biosensors

There has been a substantial amount of research into ways to incorporate whole cells, pieces of cells, or subcellular elements from bacteria, plants, and animals into biosensors while maintaining their natural biological or biochemical functions. Unique combinations of enzymes or highly sensitive physiological receptor mechanisms that are present in intact cells or tissues may be impossible to duplicate using isolated enzymes in the biosensor. It is also conceivable that living organisms could provide inexpensive sources for bioselective materials used in biosensors. Despite some successful research with various biological elements from intact tissues described in the following section, "living" biosensors have not been as widely explored as other types of biosensors and may be perceived as having fewer commercial applications.

9.1 MICROBIAL BIOSENSORS

Living microorganisms (algae, bacteria, yeast, and fungi) can be used as the biocatalytic element for biosensors, as illustrated in Figure 9.1. A wide range of potential analytes is possible, since different microorganisms have their own, unique complement of biochemical activities. Microbial biosensors might be simpler and less expensive to develop for some applications, eliminating the need for isolation and purification of enzymes and related cofactors that are required for an enzyme-based biosensor. However, a microbial biosensor using a microorganism that has a wide range of biochemical activities could be disadvantageous, since it might not have the highly specific selectivity to a particular chemical substrate that would be possible with a biosensor based on an isolated, purified enzyme. On the

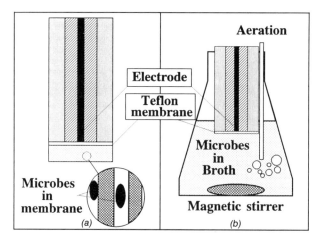

FIGURE 9.1. *Two modes of operation for a microbial biosensor using an electrochemical transducer. (a) The microbes are immobilized within a membrane on the biosensor. (b) The microbes are cultured in an aerated broth in which the biosensor is immersed.*

other hand, the diverse biochemistry of living microbes could be advantageous in some cases. Microbes can respond to complex mixtures of chemicals, and microbial biosensors have been developed for screening mutagens or for evaluating the effectiveness of wastewater treatment procedures, as discussed further on. It may not be possible to develop a biosensor using several isolated enzymes for applications where multiple chemical species must be detected. Microbial biosensors might be able to accomplish this feat, but may also require more careful attention than enzyme-based biosensors. A microbial biosensor must be provided with appropriate nutrients and a favorable environment so that the microorganisms can remain alive and viable. The biosensor must be carefully stored in order to remain sensitive for long time periods. If the biosensor is exposed to chemical species that are toxic to these microorganisms, there will be a corresponding loss in sensitivity as the cells die. However, since it is relatively easy to grow the microorganisms in cell cultures, there would be adequate material to replenish the biosensor.

9.1.1 Immobilization Methods

A microbial biosensor must include some mechanism for immobilizing the microbes next to the sensing transducer, for example as shown in Figure 9.1(a). Also, the sensor must be covered with a semipermeable membrane that allows the chemical species of interest to cross the membrane while retaining microbes within the biosensor. Oxygen and other necessary nutrients must also be free to diffuse into the biosensor to maintain aerobic conditions for the microbes. The simplest method for immobilization is to centrifuge or filter a microbial suspension onto a supporting membrane. Filter paper, nylon sheets, acetylcellulose, and dialysis membranes have been used for this purpose. Pores within the membrane material entrap the microbes, providing a mechanical support. The physical dimensions of the microbes and the thickness of the membrane influence the time response for the sensor. Alternately, an immobilizing layer of gel can be used. Agar, gelatin, collagen, polyacrylamide, and polyvinylalcohol gels have been successfully used in microbial sensors, although biosensor time responses invariably become slower with these gels due to diffusional limitations.

Gels formed from polyvinylalcohols appear to be the most promising and provide the mildest conditions for immobilization. Renneberg et al. (1988) reported that polyvinylalcohol gels have very good O_2 permeability and diffusivity. Polyvinylalcohols modified by stilbazolium groups, which are polymerized by illumination with visible light, may be more suitable than gels that are polymerized by UV light. Free radicals generated during polymerization by UV light might be harmful to the microbes. Apparently, there has not been much success using chemical methods for immobilizing microbes by the covalent or other chemical binding techniques that are successful with enzymes, probably due to cell membrane damage and unacceptable losses in biological activity. An alternate method is to grow the microbes in a suspension, as shown in Figure 9.1(b).

9.1.2 Transducers

As with enzyme-based biosensors, there has been a great deal of research using conventional electrochemical transducers in microbial biosensors. Common techniques include monitoring the rate of O_2 utilization, CO_2 production, or change in pH with respiration. Metabolic products, such as H_2 and H_2S gases, H_2O_2, ammonia, and other ions can also be monitored. Both amperometric and potentiometric electrodes, as discussed previously for enzyme-based biosensors, have been successfully employed.

The first microbial biosensor, using cells of *Acetobacter xylinum*, was developed by Divies (1975) to detect ethanol. In the 15 years since then, there has been a rapid proliferation of new microbial biosensor designs, especially for fermentation and environmental applications. Riedel et al. (1989) and Malochán (1991) have recently reviewed microbial biosensors reported in the literature which have been designed to detect over 50 different chemical species. The majority of these applications are based on changes in metabolism monitored with O_2 electrodes, including detection of acetic acid, alcohols (ethanol, methanol), amino acids (L-glutamic acid, L-tryptophan), antibiotics (nystatin), carbohydrates (glucose, fructose, maltose, and sucrose), cholesterol, hydrocarbons (hexadecane, methane), nitrogenous compounds (creatinine, NH_3, NH_4^+, NO_2^-, urea, uric acid), peptides (angiotensin, aspartame, gonadotropine-releasing hormone), phenol, phosphate, and vitamins (L-ascorbic acid).

Oxygen electrodes have also been used in microbial biosensors to detect enzyme activities (α-amylase, protease). Ammonia ion–sensitive transducers have been used in microbial biosensors to detect amino acids (L-arginine, L-asparagine, L-aspartic acid, L-glutamine, L-histidine, L-tyrosine, L-serine), nicotinamide, NAD^+, nitriloacetic acid, NO_2^-, and urea. Carbon dioxide transducers have been used in microbial biosensors to detect amino acids (L-aspartic acid, L-glutamic acid, L-lysine), formic acid, glucose, pyruvate, and uric acid. Hydrogen ion (pH) sensors have been used in microbial biosensors to detect antibiotics (cephalosporins), carbohydrates (galactose, glucose, mannose), lactate, monomethyl sulfate, and nicotinic acid. A fuel cell–type H_2 gas sensor has been used in microbial biosensors to detect formic acid and sulfide. Besides electrochemical transducers, all of the other types of transducer technologies discussed in the previous chapters can also be adapted for use in microbial biosensors.

9.2 BIOLUMINESCENT BACTERIA

Luciferases are specific enzymes responsible for the ability of some living organisms to emit light. For example, marine bacteria (e.g., *Vibrio fischeri, Vibrio harveyi, Photobacterium phosphoreum, Photobacterium leiognathi*) emit visible blue-green light at rates between 10^2 to 10^4 quanta per second per cell. Luciferases catalyze the reaction between flavin, aliphatic aldehyde, and O_2

$$FMNH_2 + RCHO + O_2 \rightarrow FMN + RCOOH + H_2O + h\nu \quad (149)$$

to produce light. The O_2 molecule is split to form water and a long-chain acid product. Only aliphatic aldehydes with 8 to 18 carbon chains are effective in the previous reaction. Luciferase functions as a shunt in the respiratory electron-transport pathway, and can be coupled with NADH or NADPH through oxidoreductases that catalyze the reaction of FMN back to flavin. Although the specific mechanism(s) and the structure of the light emitter are not fully understood, the luminescent properties can be exploited for biosensors. Blum and Gautier (1991) have compiled fairly extensive tables of analytes detected with optical biosensors using either immobilized firefly luciferase or with bioluminescent enzymes derived from bacteria. Intact bacteria may be useful for the same types of measurements, and may be able to more readily maintain optimum conditions for the bioluminescent reaction compared to isolated enzyme systems.

9.3 YEAST-BASED BIOSENSORS

Kubiak and Wang (1989) described a yeast-modified carbon paste electrode that is sensitive to primary alcohols. Dry "Red Star" active yeast granules (Universal Foods, Milwaukee, WI) were mixed with graphite powder and mineral oil. Carbon pastes containing 2, 5, and 10% (w/w) yeast were tested. The modified carbon pastes were either packed into a glass tube (3 mm opening) with the amplifier connected by a copper wire or into the electrode cavity of a thin-layer flow detector. Measurements were obtained for different alcohol concentrations in the presence of 1 mM NAD^+ and potassium hexacyanoferrate(III) in a well-stirred 0.05 M phosphate buffer (pH = 7.4). Potassium hexacyanoferrate was used as a redox mediator, permitting the transfer of electrons for the oxidation of NADH to occur at a lower potential. Steady state current responses to 0.5 mM ethanol at a potential of 0.6 V were reported to be 298, 405, and 590 nA respectively for the test solutions with 2, 5 and 10% yeast contents. In the flow injection tests, the 95% response times ranged from 7 to 10 seconds.

The yeast–carbon paste electrode sensitivity and linearity were examined for different alcohols. The order of sensitivity for the following primary alcohols was: ethanol > 1-propanol > 1-butanol > 1-amyl alcohol. The electrodes were not sensitive to methanol, or to the secondary alcohols 2-propanol and 2-butanol. The current-concentration relationships were found to be nonlinear as expected for enzyme-catalyzed reactions. From double-reciprocal Lineweaver-Burk plots, the apparent Michaelis-Menten constants (K_m) were estimated to be 1.0, 1.3, and 1.4 mM respectively for ethanol, 1-butanol, and 1-propanol. The Lineweaver-Burk plot for 1-amyl alcohol was not described by simple Michaelis-Menten kinetics. For low alcohol concentrations below the apparent K_m, current-concentration relationships were approximately linear. The alcohol content of several commercial beverages, including vodka, red and white wines, and beer were measured and found to be in good agreement with the labeled values.

9.4 BOTANICAL BIOSENSORS

Plants also are sources of the enzymes needed for specific biosensors. It may be possible to extract these enzymes less expensively than by genetic engineering or by other, more elaborate biochemical processing techniques. A wide variety of biosensors have been tested using enzymes from plants.

Rechnitz (1981) described a glutamic acid biosensor using a thin slice of yellow squash removed from the mesocarp layer, which is directly under the outer skin. Glutamic acid is used as a seasoning for foods. The yellow squash plant tissue is a good source of glutamate decarboxylase, which produces CO_2 gas in the reaction with glutamic acid. A CO_2 transducer based on a pH electrode was used.

Botré et al. (1991) used a potato, thinly sliced (100 μm) by a microtome knife, for a catechol biosensor. The potato contained polyphenol oxidase. The slice was soaked in a pH 6.6 bis-Tris-0.1 M HCl solution for two hours to remove phenols, then was placed over the gas-permeable membrane of a Clark O_2 electrode. The top surface of the potato slice was covered with a dialysis membrane. The O_2 evolution in response to catechol, dopamine, L-dopa, adrenalin, noradrenalin, ascorbic acid, and glucose was tested. The biosensor was linear in the range from 25 to 230 μM catechol. The biosensor was found to have an initially rapid response, with a secondary, slower response, probably due to the relatively large diffusion distances required for a thick slice. The selectivity of the biosensor to the other compounds measured after four and six minutes was compared to the catechol responses. Dopamine had the largest interference, 15% after four minutes and 70% after six minutes compared to the catechol response. The corresponding responses were 10% at four minutes and 45% at six minutes for L-dopa. Ascorbic acid had 20% interference, while adrenalin and noradrenalin responses were only about 5%. Glucose had no effect. The lifetime of the biosensor was two to three months, with roughly 20% loss in sensitivity over the first two weeks.

Uchiyama and Umetsu (1991) recently described a biosensor for L-ascorbic acid that uses cucumber juice. The juice was prepared by homogenizing cucumber in a phosphate buffer at pH = 7.0, followed by filtration through a 0.2 μm pore filter to remove the plant pulp. The juice also contained 0.1% sodium azide, which was added as a stabilizing agent. A concentrated juice fraction was then extracted after centrifugation at 3,000 r.p.m. for 20 minutes. The separated fraction contained ascorbate oxidase, which catalyzes the reaction

$$\text{L-ascorbic acid} + \frac{1}{2}O_2 \xrightarrow{\text{ascorbate oxidase}} \text{dehydroascorbic acid} + H_2O \qquad (150)$$

A 150 μL volume of the concentrated cucumber juice was allowed to soak into a 0.2 mm thick, 5 mm diameter porous felt pad. This pad was placed over the gas-permeable membrane of a Clark O_2 electrode, with the top surface of the felt pad open to the atmosphere. The transient evolution of O_2 was monitored after adding a 5 μL drop of distilled water containing different concentrations of ascorbic acid. The sensor was found to be linear in the concentration range from 0.25 to 1.6 mM, but became nonlinear at higher concentrations. The sensitivity of the O_2 electrode was 0.33 μamp/mM ascorbic acid in the linear range. The effect of the sodium azide preservative on the peak current was also investigated. At the 0.1% concentration used, the peak current was depressed by about 50% compared to pure juice. Higher sodium azide concentrations further depressed the maximum current peak. The biosensor was found to have a lifetime of about two weeks when stored at 4°C. Strawberry and orange juices were also tested, and were also found to provide sources of ascorbate oxidase for the biosensor reaction.

Malochán (1991) has compiled a table of some other biosensors using botanical materials. These include banana pulp for detecting dopamine and oxalate, carnation flower homogenate for detecting urea, chrysanthemum flower receptacles for detecting some amino acids, jack bean meal for detecting urea, mushrooms for detecting mono- and polyphenols, and sugar beet for detecting L-tyrosine. Many other possibilities for botanically based biosensors exist.

9.5 BIOSENSORS USING CULTURED CELLS

9.5.1 Biosensors Using pH Measurements

The LAPS silicone semiconductor device, described previously in Chapter 6, can be used with different types of cultured animal cells to monitor toxic effects from xenobiotics, for metabolic and signal transduction studies, or for pharmaceutical testing. The LAPS Cytosensor™ (Molecular Devices Corporation, Menlo Park, CA) is shown schematically in Figure 9.2. Each sensor chip contains a very small flow chamber, 100 μm deep and 6 mm in diameter, with a volume of only 3 μL. The microphysiometer has a total of eight chambers where either adherent or nonadherent cells can be cultured and monitored. Adherent cells can be grown on a glass cover slip, which is then transferred to cover the microphysiometer chamber. Only a relatively small number of cells, between 10^4 to 10^6, need to be cultured. When nonadherent cells are used, additional microfabrication techniques are required to modify the surface of the LAPS sensor. Nonadherent cells can be trapped in these wells by introducing a suspension of cells, then

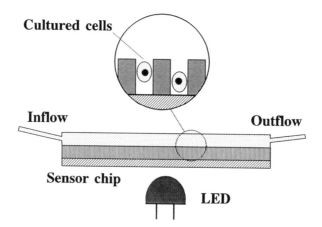

FIGURE 9.2. *Light-addressable, pH-sensitive silicon chip is used in microphysiometer design (Cytosensor™, Molecular Devices Corporation) with cultured cells and other biological samples to determine acidification rates when flow is stopped, or with other biochemical stimuli.*

slowing or stopping flow to allow sedimentation. By adjusting the nutrient flow rate, excess cells are washed out and the trapped cells remain in the microphysiometer. After cells are loaded, the nutrient flow (typically between 50 to 100 μL/minute) is interrupted at periodic intervals. During stopped flow, the rate of acidification (dpH/dt) can be measured with a precision on the order of 0.01 pH units. Different conditions tested so far have elicited 10 to 200% changes in the acidification rate. After a series of measurements is completed, the cells can be washed out using high flow rates, and new cells can be introduced into the microphysiometer for further testing.

Parce et al. (1989) used the LAPS microphysiometer to test various stimuli with murine fibroblasts and with human epidermal keratinocytes, bathed in Dulbecco's modified Eagles's medium with 10% fetal bovine serum. A confluent layer, equivalent to approximately 10^7 cells/mm^3, caused changes in potential ranging from 2 to 100 μV/second, or roughly from 0.002 to 0.098 pH units/minute. A metabolic uncoupler, carbonylcyanide chlorophenylhydrazone, which stimulates mitochondrial O_2 uptake, was found to double dpH/dt. The time rate of recovery could be followed, taking about 20 minutes for dpH/dt to return back to control after washing out the metabolic uncoupler. The stimulatory effect of epidermal growth factor on human keratinocytes was demonstrated, showing an increase in dpH/dt at concentrations as low as 0.1 ng/mL. At 10 ng/mL, a doubling of dpH/dt was seen within five minutes, presumably due to a similar increase in metabolic activity of the cells within the chamber. An adaptive response, where dpH/dt declined back towards control somewhat, was also seen.

Cytotoxicity studies were also performed with two tumor cell lines that were either resistant or sensitive to drugs. In these studies, the metabolic activity could be followed for over 24 hours. The irritancy of several chemicals was evaluated using cultured keratinocytes. The volume fraction of irritant sufficient to reduce dpH/dt by 50% (MRD_{50}) was extrapolated from dose-response studies. The values for $\log_{10}(MRD_{50})$ with a severe irritant, benzalkonium chloride, was >4 while a mild irritant, propylene glycol, was <0.5. Other moderate irritants tested were between these values. Parce et al. (1989) concluded that the LAPS-based microphysiometer can provide a sensitive and accurate bioassay for changes in metabolic activity in response to a wide variety of stimuli. For example, receptor-mediated bioassays, including those used in screening for new therapeutic drugs, are possible and preliminary studies have been completed. Signal transduction, agonist and antagonist profiles, growth factor responses, and cytokine/lymphokine responses have also been studied with the LAPS microphysiometer. Toxicology studies using various cell types with the microphysiometer would appear to be a viable alternative to the Draize (rabbit eye) test.

9.5.2 Biosensors Using Piezoelectric Microbalance

Ebersole et al. (1991) described another type of microphysiometer that uses a piezoelectric transducer to detect changes in mass on its surface (Chapter 6). A quartz crystal with a 0.35 cm² gold electrode on one side was used as the mass detecting element. The change in mass was caused by the attachment of a pH-sensitive polymer to the surface. The positive or negative ionic charge of the polymer changes with pH and determines its solubility in cell culture solutions. The polymer solubility reaches a minimum at the isoelectric point, which occurs when the pH is around 6.14, and the polymer can precipitate out of solution. The isoelectric point can be manipulated by changing the composition of the different monomers that are used in making the polymer. At higher or lower pH, the solubility increases. As the pH of the solution causes the polymer solubility to decrease, the polymer starts to adhere to the gold surface of the piezoelectric transducer. Changes in mass can be detected over a wide pH range, well before visible precipitation of the polymer is observed.

Ebersol et al. (1991) used this device to measure the growth rates of *Escherichia coli* and *Staphylococcus aureus* cultures with different initial cell densities, various nutrient compositions, and in the presence of antibiotics to inhibit growth. The rate of growth is related to the rate of acidification (dpH/dt), which can be measured by the piezoelectric sensor, since the mass change due to polymer attachment is related to pH. Samples with very low cell densities (5,000 cells/mL) could produce measurable changes after four hours. The device is reusable, since the sensor surface can be easily renewed by washing with acidic or basic solution that increases the polymer solubility. Although this sensor has not yet been tested with mammalian cells, it may be useful for the same types of studies proposed previously for the LAPS microphysiometer, provided that the polymer does not adversely affect the metabolism of the cultured cells.

9.5.3 Biosensors Using Calorimetric Measurements

The small calorimetric vessel designed by Bäckman and Wadsö (1991), shown previously in Figure 7.1, was tested using cultures of human T-lymphoma cells and with cultures of *Escherichia coli*. This system also allows O_2 consumption and acidification rates (dpH/dt) to be measured with conventional electrochemical transducers by stopping nutrient flow through the sample chamber for short time periods.

9.6 BIOSENSORS USING INTACT TISSUES

In a review written for *Science* over 10 years ago, Rechnitz (1981) included descriptions for some examples of biosensors that he had developed using slices of animal tissues as the bioselective element. This included a biosensor for glutamine using a 0.5 mm slice of cortical tissue from the pig kidney, placed over an ammonia-sensitive electrode. Rechnitz and co-workers received a U.S. patent (#4,216,065) for this biosensor in 1980. He reported that the kidney tissue could be stored for several months at 4°C without loss of activity. In phosphate buffer at pH 7.8, the biosensor sensitivity was 50 mV per decade of glutamine concentration in the range from 6×10^{-5} to 6.7×10^{-3} M, with a lower limit of detection of 2×10^{-5} M and response time around five to seven minutes. He reported that there were negligible interferences from L-alanine, L-arginine, L-histidine, L-valine, L-serine, L-glutamic acid, L-aspartic acid, D-alanine, D-aspartic acid, glycine, or creatinine. He also reported that the lifetime of the animal tissue–based sensor could be extended to around thirty days by adding 0.02% sodium azide preservative to inhibit bacterial growth. Budantsev (1991) described a biosensor for catecholamines using rat liver slices. The tissue was frozen and cut into 25 to 200 μm thick slices, then was placed on a nylon mesh and allowed to dry in air. An ammonia transducer was used to detect catecholamines from the reaction

monoamine oxidase

$$RCH_2NH_2 \rightarrow RCHO + NH_3 \qquad (151)$$

where the enzyme monoamine oxidase, which is normally bound on the internal membranes of living mitochondria, must have retained its activity in the treated tissue. Malochan (1991) has compiled a table of some other biosensors using animal tissues, including mouse intestinal mucosa to detect adenosine, rabbit muscle to detect adenosine 5' monophosphate, and rabbit liver to detect guanine.

9.6.1 Neuronal Biosensors

Unique, chemosensitive biosensors have been developed using neuronal receptors. Buch and Rechnitz (1989) reviewed research with antennae removed from blue crabs, which have specialized chemosensory cells. These receptors allow the animal to locate food. Sensitivities to analytes such as glutamic acid, isoleucine, and other amino acids, and to purines (adenine and adenosine nucleotides) can be monitored from the changes in frequency for action potentials that are generated and sent out through different nerves. For example, Wijesuriya and Rechnitz (1992) recently described a neuronal biosensor that uses a crayfish antenna as the active element, as shown schematically in Figure 9.3. The antenna was dissected free and a sensory nerve exposed. The nerve was impaled with a glass microelectrode filled with physiological salt solution for standard neurological recording of nerve activity spikes in response to chemosensory stimulation. The sensitivity of this neuronal biosensor to pyrazinamide, a drug used for tuberculosis treatment, was tested. This drug is damaging to the human liver at concentrations > 35 mg/kg and has been associated with patient deaths. The frequency of spikes was recorded over a concentration range from 10^{-10} to 10^{-3} M. A very nonlinear curve was generated, reaching a maximum firing frequency around 150 spikes/second at concentrations $> 10^{-4}$ M. An approximately linear region was found in the range from 10^{-5} to 10^{-4} M, with the firing frequency increasing from about 30 to 80 spikes/second. The biosensor was not sensitive to 15 other compounds tested, including essential amino acids, excitatory amino acids, neurotransmitters, alcohols, hormones, and sugars. The lifetime of the "living biosensor" was only 8 to 10 hours when tested with 1 mM pyrazinamide

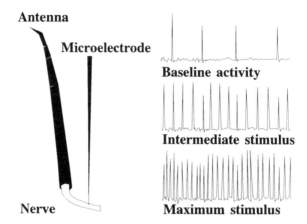

FIGURE 9.3. *Example of a biological element with chemosensory transduction: the antenna of the crayfish. Neural discharge increases with the concentration of the analyte.*

doses every hour, which evoked close to the maximum chemoreceptor responses. The lifetime was even shorter with higher doses.

9.6.2 Single Cell Secretory Events

Recently, Wightman et al. (1991) have reported the first studies of catecholamine secretion from individual secretory vesicles in cultured bovine medullary chromaffin cells. Beveled carbon fiber microelectrodes were placed very close to individual cells, which were then stimulated with various chemical substances including nicotine, carbamoylcholine, and elevated potassium. Mechanical stimuli were also presented to the cells. The carbon fiber microelectrode was operated in an amperometric mode, polarized at +0.65 V relative to a saturated calomel electrode to oxidize catecholamines. Current spikes were seen with the chemical and mechanical stimuli, which could be completely eliminated by removing Ca^{2+} ions from the cell culture medium.

Wightman et al. (1991) demonstrated that the current spikes were due to the oxidation of catecholamines released from single vesicles, which have average diameters around 156 nm. The charge was calculated from the area underneath each current spike, after subtracting a baseline secretion envelope due to the accumulation of catecholamine released from other nearby vesicles. The charge was constant, around 1×10^{-12} coulomb, and was not a function of the chemical stimulus. This would be expected since each vesicle releases essentially a fixed volume of catecholamines. The concentration of catecholamine released by a single vesicle was estimated to be about 5 attomoles, consistent with other calculated estimates in the literature. The frequency of vesicle release was found to be greater with the stronger stimuli, which is also consistent with theoretical expectations.

A later study by Chow et al. (1992) has been conducted with isolated, cultured bovine chromaffin cells using a similar experimental technique with carbon fiber microelectrodes. In their study, they impaled cells with an electrolyte-filled glass microelectrode and used voltage clamp techniques to depolarize and excite the cell. A carbon fiber microelectrode, polarized at +0.8 V, was placed near the cell to detect catecholamine release from the vesicles. They were also able to follow changes in the cell membrane capacitance through the glass microelectrode. They observed short time delays after excitation before secretory release, and also saw a small rise in catecholamines before vesicle release. This latter effect may be due to catecholamines leaking through a small opening before the vesicle completely dumps out its contents.

9.7 BIOSENSORS USING RECEPTOR ELEMENTS

9.7.1 Membrane Receptors

It may be possible to incorporate the receptor elements directly into a biosensor, if the receptor elements can be isolated and retain their function. Wingard (1990) has reviewed research based on this concept. Two major receptor types, based either on ion channels or on secondary messenger systems, may be useful. The opening and closing of individual channels in the receptor membrane in response to analytes could be monitored using patch-clamp microelectrodes. Another technique that has been investigated is to attach the receptor to the gate of an FET. DNA expression research is presently directed towards studies of receptor proteins, but could be used to produce adequate receptor proteins for use in biosensors.

9.7.2 Nicotinic Acetylcholine Receptor Biosensor

For example, Rogers et al. (1992) coupled the LAPS microphysiometer with nicotinic acetylcholine receptors isolated from the electric organ of the *Torpedo californica* electric eel (Biofish Associates, Georgetown, MA). The acetylcholine receptor was fluorescent-labeled with carboxyfluorescein-*N*-hydroxysuccinimide (Molecular Devices, Menlo Park, CA), although the fluorescence was not studied. The label provided a binding site for recognition by an antibody, as described in the following. A nitrocellulose filter membrane was incubated with biotin, streptavidin, and α-bungarotoxin (Molecular Probes, Eugene, OR). Then the labeled nicotinic acetylcholine receptors were immobilized by forming a complex with the biotin and streptavidin during slow filtration through the membrane. Excess materials were washed away with more rapid filtration. The amount of remaining complex was quantified using an antibody and enzyme conjugate, antifluorescein-IgG-urease. The antibody attached to the fluorescein label on the receptor. Reversible binding occurs between the receptor and α-bungarotoxin, which can be displaced by other ligands. In the presence of a known concentration of urea, a pH change occurs as a result of the NH_4^+ formed from the urease-catalyzed hydrolysis reaction [Equation (92)] that can be measured by the LAPS transducer.

Well-known receptor agonists including acetylcholine, carbamylcholine, and nicotine, and receptor antagonists, including α-bungarotoxin, Naja toxin (a snake venom), and d-tubocurarine, were used to test the biosensor. The ligand concentration that inhibited the biosensor response by 50% (IC_{50}) was determined, and this value was used to calculate the apparent binding affinity for each ligand. The affinities for these agonists and antagonists were compared to literature values obtained by radioisotope binding assays, and for some previously reported fiberoptic biosensor studies. The binding affinities were similar to the radioisotope values. The nicotinic acetylcholine receptor modified LAPS biosensor was reported to be more sensitive than fiberoptic biosensors, by several orders of magnitude in some cases.

9.8 REFERENCES

Bäckman, P. and I. Wadsö. 1991. "Cell Growth Experiments Using a Microcalorimetric Vessel Equipped with Oxygen and pH Electrodes," *J. Biochem. Biophys. Meth.*, 23:283–293.

Botré, F., F. Mazzei, M. Lanzi, G. Lorenti and C. Botré. 1991. "Plant-Tissue Electrode for the Determination of Catechol," *Anal. Chim. Acta*, 255:59–62.

Buch, R. M. and G. A. Rechnitz. 1989. "Neuronal Biosensors," *Anal. Chem.*, 61:533A–542A.

Budantsev, A. Y. 1991. "Biosensor for Catecholamines with Immobilized Monoamine Oxidase in Tissue Sections," *Anal. Chim. Acta*, 249:71–76.

Chow, R. H., L. von Rüden and E. Neher. 1992. "Delay in Vesicle Fusion Revealed by Electrochemical Monitoring of Single Secretory Events in Adrenal Chromaffin Cells," *Nature*, 356:60–63.

Divies, C. 1975. "Ethanol Oxidation by an Acetobacter Xylinum Microbial Electrode," *Ann. Microbiol. (Paris)*, 126A:175–186.

Ebersole, R. C., R. P. Foss and M. D. Ward. 1991. "Piezoelectric Cell Growth Sensor," *Bio/Technol.*, 9:450–454.

Kubiak, W. W. and J. Wang. 1989. "Yeast-Based Carbon Paste Bioelectrode for Ethanol," *Anal. Chim. Acta*, 221:43–51.

Macholán, L. 1991. "Biocatalytic Membrane Electrodes," in *Bioinstrumentation and Biosensors*, D. L. Wise, ed., New York, NY: M. Dekker, Inc., pp. 329–378.

Parce, J. W., J. C. Owicki, K. M. Kercso, G. B. Sigal, H. G. Wada, V. C. Muir, L. J. Bousse, K. L. Ross, B. R. Sikic and H. M. McConnell. 1989. "Detection of Cell-Affecting Agents with a Silicon Biosensor," *Science Wash. DC*, 246:243–247.

Rechnitz, G. A. 1981. "Bioselective Membrane Electrode Probes," *Science Wash. DC*, 214:287–291.

Renneberg, R., K. Sonomoto, S. Katoh and A. Tanaka. 1988. "Oxygen Diffusivity of Synthetic Gels Derived from Prepolymers," *Appl. Microbiol. Biotechn.*, 28:1–7.

Riedel, K., R. Renneberg, U. Wollenberger, G. Kaiser and F. W. Scheller. 1989. "Microbial Sensors: Fundamentals and Application for Process Control," *J. Chem. Tech Biotechnol.*, 44:85–106.

Rogers, K. R., J. C. Fernando, R. G. Thompson, J. J. Valdes and M. E. Eldefrawi. 1992. "Detection of Nicotinic Receptor Ligands with a Light Addressable Potentiometric Sensor," *Anal. Biochem.*, 202:111–116.

Uchiyama, S. and U. Umetsu. 1991. "Concentration-Step Amperometric Sensor of L-Ascorbic Acid Using Cucumber Juice," *Anal. Chim. Acta*, 255:53–58.

Wightman, R. M., J. A. Jankowski, R. T. Kennedy, K. T. Kawsagoe, T. J. Schroeder, D. J. Leszczyszyn, J. A. Near, E. J. Diliberto, Jr. and O. H. Viveros. 1991. "Temporally Resolved Catecholamine Spikes Correspond to Single Vesicle Release from Individual Chromaffin Cells," *Proc. Natl. Acad. Sci. USA*, 88:10754–10758.

Wijesuriya, D. and G. A. Rechnitz. 1992. "Construction and Properties of a Pyrazinamide-Selective Biosensor Using Chemoreceptor Structures from Crayfish," *Anal. Chim. Acta*, 256:39–46.

Wingard, L. B., Jr. 1990. "Biosensor Trends. Receptors, Enzymes, and Antibodies," in *Enzyme Engineering—10*, H. Okada, A. Tanaka and H. W. Blanch, eds., *Annals N.Y. Acad. Sci.*, 613:44–53.

CHAPTER 10

Future Directions

10.1 SCANNING ELECTROCHEMICAL MICROSCOPY

Extremely fine probes have already been developed which can be used to map out extremely detailed surface features. A three-dimensional representation of a region can be made by systematically sweeping the probe (scanning) across the sample. Here, "scanning" refers to a physical movement, and not the time-dependent change in potential or current as has been used for electrochemical scans referred to in the previous chapters. Scanning tunneling microscopy, for example, uses the electron tunneling current through a fine probe to obtain measurements at the atomic level.

Bard et al. (1991) have developed a scanning electrochemical microscope. The fine tip of an electrochemical transducer is moved in nanometer increments by a computer-controlled piezoelectric translation element to scan a region. Of course there are practical limitations on how close the probe can be placed to a surface, particularly when the surface is irregular or is moving. Vibration of the sample or of the mechanical apparatus holding the probe can also be a limiting factor. The resolution of the electrochemical microscope depends on the diameter of the scanning tip and the distance from the tip to the sample. As with any other electrochemical transducer, the time response depends on diffusion, convective mass transfer, and the kinetics of the chemical reactions that occur at the scanning tip for all of the chemical species involved.

10.1.1 Conductivity Measurements

The simplest type of measurement with this system is the change in current over surfaces that have variations in electrical conductivity. For example, the current above an interdigitated electrode array was measured by Bard et al. (1991). The array consisted of alternating 3 μm wide bands of Pt separated by 5 μm spaces of SiO_2 substrate. The electrode array was covered with an electrically conducting solution and scanned with a glass-coated 0.2 μm diameter Pt electrode held at a negative potential relative to a calomel reference electrode. The current increased sharply over the conducting Pt bands, and dropped to very low levels over the insulating bands of SiO_2. The resulting electrochemical scans could be represented either as a three-dimensional composite plot, or as a two-dimensional gray scale plot by displaying the magnitude of the current as a relative intensity. This method could be used to map out the surface features of electronic devices and identify possible defects.

10.1.2 Enzyme Kinetic Measurements

In a similar manner, the reactions catalyzed by enzymes can be studied with biosensors as they are moved past a biological surface by physical scanning techniques. Preliminary results for the kinetics of glucose oxidase were presented by Bard et al. (1991). Current gradients were measured above a nylon membrane bound with glucose oxidase, using an 8 μm diameter carbon fiber microelectrode in the presence of the redox mediator ferrocene-carboxylic acid. Measurements were made with and without glucose, with the electrode polarized at +0.6 V. The gradient above the membrane was found to be much steeper in the presence of glucose, and the forward rate constant for an irreversible surface reaction was determined to be $k_f = 1.89 \times 10^{-3}$ cm/sec.

The scanning electrochemical microscope was also used by Bard et al. (1991) to study the surfaces of isolated mitochondria, which have very small dimensions ranging from 0.5 to 3 μm. Information on the heterogeneity of surface properties of biological samples and the kinetics of various types of biochemical reactions could be obtained by nondestructive electrochemical measurements using the tip scanning technique.

10.1.3 Oxygen Gradient Studies

The author has used similar types of spatially detailed electrochemical scanning by controlling the movement of Whalen-Nair type recessed cathode PO_2 microelectrodes with tip diameters <2 μm (Chapter 5) with 1 μm step resolution micropositioners. For example, spatially detailed tissue PO_2 gradients have been measured in brain and liver slices (Buerk and Saidel, 1978), across blood vessel walls *in vivo* (Buerk and Goldstick, 1982) and across thin layers of hemoglobin and myoglobin solutions (Buerk et al.,

1989). In the first study, the metabolic rate and K_m were determined by optimizing the computer-generated curve fit to the Michaelis-Menten model. Other metabolic models that had analytical solutions were also directly curve fit to the data, but the Michaelis-Menten model gave the best match to the experimental measurements. In the last study, model parameters for the oxyhemoglobin and myoglobin saturation curves could be obtained by fitting the data. For example, the P_{50} for myoglobin was found to be 1.26 Torr (0.168 kPa) at room temperature.

In a recent study, *in vivo* PO_2 gradients were measured in the vitreous humor around arterioles and venules in the cat eye (Buerk et al., in press), as shown schematically in Figure 10.1 A PO_2 microelectrode was positioned using a pivoting microdrive system designed by Pournaras et al. (1991). By moving the microelectrode over different retinal vessels, spatially detailed PO_2 gradients were measured in the aqueous humor above the retina. A simple radial diffusion model was fit to the data and the O_2 flux was calculated for each vessel studied. For the example shown in Figure 10.1, measurements were made near a parallel arteriole and venule pair, which were carrying blood in a countercurrent direction. There was a drop

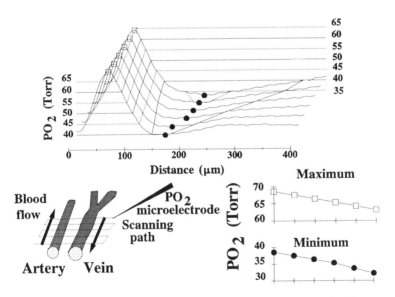

FIGURE 10.1. *Example of electrochemical scanning technique applied to O_2 measurements over a pair of blood vessels in the retina of a cat eye (left corner). The choice of scanning path in the vitreous humor above the vessels determines the spatial variation in PO_2 (top). The artery is leaking O_2 out into the vitreous humor, while the vein is picking up O_2. Maximum (squares) and minimum (circles) values are indicated (bottom right).*

in the maximum PO_2 above the arteriole as the microelectrode was moved downstream.

All of the arterioles investigated in this study were losing O_2, although the amount of O_2 loss was quite small compared to the total amount of O_2 carried as oxyhemoglobin in the flowing blood. At this location, O_2 was diffusing into the venule, and the minimum PO_2 appeared to be increasing in the direction of venous blood flow. This suggested that O_2 was being picked up (diffusional shunting) from the external environment by the venous blood. Not all venules were gaining O_2 in these cat eye experiments. In other *in vivo* eye experiments in progress, PO_2 and K^+ ion-sensitive microelectrodes are being used in concert with a laser Doppler method to measure blood flow in the cat optic nerve head (Buerk et al., 1992). Highly localized changes in chemical environment and blood flow are being measured in response to flickering light stimuli delivered to the eye at various frequencies.

The author also has another PO_2 microelectrode gradient study in progress using cultured bovine retinal epithelium cells (Buerk and Khatami, unpublished). From the steepness of the measured PO_2 gradients in the culture medium above the cells, the metabolic rate for the confluent monolayer of cells can be determined. Differences in O_2 metabolism after adding adenosine and other chemical substrates are presently being quantified by this technique.

The physical scanning technique can be combined with other types of microelectrodes, electrochemical transducers, or biosensors as long as they have sufficiently small tip dimensions. It may be possible to spatially map multiple analytes with multibarrel microelectrodes. Pulse voltammetry techniques can also be used to measure more than one chemical species with a single microelectrode by examining the individual redox potentials for each analyte. In addition to chemical concentrations, the transient measurements can be used to derive other information about the sample. For example, a chronoamperometric technique has been used by the author to measure spatial variations for the O_2 diffusion coefficient in different parts of dog and rabbit blood vessel walls (Buerk and Goldstick, in press). Roh et al. (1990) used the same technique to measure O_2 diffusion coefficients in cornea, aqueous humor, and retinal tissue of the cat eye.

10.2 NANOFABRICATION

The tools for constructing extremely small mechanical and semiconductor structures, combining computer-aided design with microlithography apparatus, etching chambers, vapor deposition, and other equipment are in place at several facilities, including the National Nanofabrication Facility at Cornell University, the Quantum Electronic Science and Technology Center at the University of California, Santa Barbara, and the Berkley Sensor and Actuator Center at the University of California, Berkley. According to a series of articles in a recent issue of *Science* magazine (November 29, 1991), both American and Japanese corporations are moving rapidly towards implementation of nanofabrication technology. Electronic circuits, previously thought to be limited to 0.1 μm (100 nanometer) dimensions, are rapidly approaching the optimum densities possible with current microlithography technology. With nanofabrication technology, circuit dimensions may soon be reduced to such small levels that they would be capable of manipulating single electrons. Focused ion-beam tools can reliably fashion features smaller than 25 nanometers (under 250 Å). Such devices may be able to increase the computing power of today's best silicon chips by perhaps three orders of magnitude. Hand-held supercomputers may be possible in the near future. This technology can be readily applied to the development of smart biosensors, as illustrated in Figure 10.2, with onboard processing to fully interpret the measurement and to precisely control the movements of calibration and sample fluids through the device.

Biological-based nanomachines are already being researched. Ferritin, an eight-nanometer wide protein from liver, has been investigated by Stephen Mann and colleagues at the University of Bath. The protein can cage (trap) molecules, such as iron oxide, manganese oxide, and iron sulfide. Ferritin performs this function to protect the body from the toxic

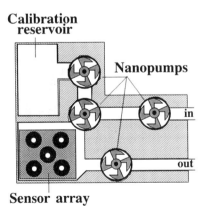

FIGURE 10.2. *Possible miniaturized multichannel biosensor using micromachined nanopumps to control fluid delivery to the sensing transducers, including capability for self-calibration.*

effects of iron oxide, and participates in the physiological recycling of iron. It may be possible to synthesize proteins that specifically cage other molecules. Such designer proteins could be linked to electronic circuits or to biosensors, and could be useful for small diagnostic machines (nanorobots) injected into the bloodstream. Nanorobots might be programmed to recognize a target organ and release drugs at the site, perform microsurgery to open up clogged atherosclerotic arteries, or perform other site-specific repairs.

10.3 MICRODIALYSIS WITH ELECTROCHEMICAL DETECTION

Implantable microdialysis probes have already been developed for monitoring different biological substrates after placing the devices into living tissues or directly into the bloodstream. A schematic drawing of the microdialysis probe is shown in Figure 10.3. A dialysis fluid is pumped through the stainless steel probe past a semipermeable membrane at flow rates usually in the 0.5 to 2 μL/minute range. Biochemical species with relatively low molecular weights are able to diffuse across the membrane into the di-

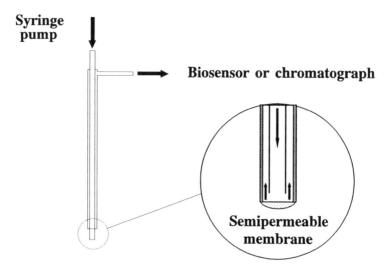

FIGURE 10.3. *Schematic drawing of microdialysis probe with outflow fluid monitored by a biosensor or by a high-performance liquid chromatograph. The probe can be implanted into the brain or other organs to monitor specific biochemical substrates, or for delivery of drugs. Concentrations of substrates crossing the semipermeable dialysis membrane depend on their concentration in tissue and the fluid flow rate through the probe.*

alyzing fluid. The dialysis fluid exiting the probe is then collected for further analysis by spectrophotometry, or by other types of chemical sensing. Neurochemical events and the pharmacokinetics of drugs have already been studied with this technology. Measurements have been made in awake, freely moving animals. These membranes exclude larger molecular weight species, so it is not possible to collect heavier proteins. The probes are still relatively large (0.2 to 0.5 mm) compared to cellular structures, and can cause tissue damage. They are also not able to maintain their permeability for long periods yet, especially when scar tissue or other inflammatory processes create diffusion barriers over the membrane. Further advances in miniaturization and advances in membrane technology and biocompatibility will surely improve these types of probes. Future applications using biosensors along with high-performance liquid chromatography to measure analytes in the effluent would be a logical extension. Besides potential medical applications, the combination of microdialysis, HPLC, and biosensor technology could be used in the food processing industries or in biotechnological applications.

10.4 ADVANCES IN SEMICONDUCTOR FABRICATION TECHNOLOGY

As discussed in Chapter 5, advances have been made combining reactive ion beam etching with photolithography to produce smaller microstructures. In addition to the possibility of constructing multiple types of transducers at very small sites, multiple species could be detected by innovative electrochemical methods. For example, Aoki et al. (1992) recently described a multichannel flow through system, which is shown schematically in Figure 10.4. A 16 channel interdigitated gold band electrode array was constructed by photolithography. Each gold band was 0.1 mm wide and 3 mm long, spaced apart evenly by 0.1 mm. The bands were exposed in a flow channel with dimensions 4 mm × 12 mm × 0.1 mm, for a total volume of 4.8 μL. Two modes of operation were tested. In the simplest mode, each band was polarized at a constant, but different voltage. The increment between voltages was equally divided over a desired voltage range using a custom-made multipotentiostat. An Ag/AgCl reference electrode was placed in the outflow line, and a glassy carbon disk auxiliary electrode was placed on the upper surface of the flow chamber. The current for each electrode was monitored as a function of time as substrate flowed through the device. It was necessary to correct the currents measured from individual electrodes for slight differences in the exposed area. Using this technique with a computer-controlled data acquisition system, a sixteen-point voltammogram, shown by a hypothetical graph in upper right of Figure

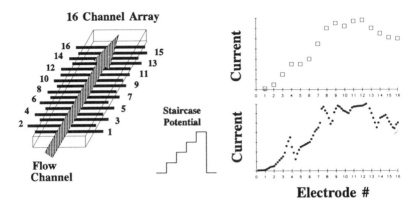

FIGURE 10.4. *Multichannel flow-through electrochemical detector developed by Aoki et al. (1992). Each gold band electrode is held at a different steady potential over a chosen voltage range. A voltammogram can be obtained with 16 data points (open squares, upper graph). Alternately, a five-step staircase voltage is applied to each electrode and a voltammogram with 80 data points is measured (circles, lower graph).*

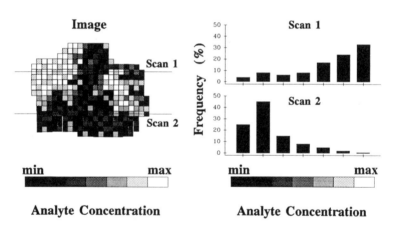

FIGURE 10.5. *Use of image processing technology for optode measurements of analyte. Intensity or light intensity changes can be measured from intracellular or intravascular locations in a noninvasive manner. By scanning specific regions (right side) and comparing with previous scans at the same location, spatial and temporal detail can be obtained.*

202

10.4, could be obtained every 14 milliseconds. Changes in the voltammogram with time could be used to detect the changes in concentration of different substrates as they flowed through the chamber.

A major advantage of this steady potential method compared to cyclic, pulse, or other time varying excitation techniques is that no charging currents are encountered. Voltammograms with much greater resolution were obtained by applying a voltage staircase with small increments to each electrode, on top of the original 16 steady voltages. With a five-step staircase changing every 37 milliseconds, a total of 80 data points could be measured at voltages in between the 16 fixed points (graph in lower right of Figure 10.4). In this case the voltammogram required 0.26 seconds. Even greater resolution could be obtained with smaller, more dense electrode arrays or with finer increments in the staircase potential.

The same concept could be applied to membrane-covered biosensors, using multichannel arrays to monitor more than one chemical species in a single sensor. Alternately, multiple sensors could be manufactured on a single surface, using masking techniques to apply specific biomembranes. The high-volume, low-cost semiconductor production techniques that are available for manufacturing these specialized ENFETs could eventually lead to much more widespread use for biosensors in which they are utilized.

10.5 ADVANCES IN OPTICAL AND IMAGING TECHNOLOGY

10.5.1 Ultra-High Resolution Light Detection

Recent advances in electronics have been continually improving the dynamic range of optical detectors. Modern computer systems are able to sample the output from light detectors at increasingly faster rates, and are able to control the excitation inputs to optical devices. Television cameras with cooled charge–coupled devices (CCDs) using silicon-integrated circuits can be used for light detection at higher sensitivities and lower cost than some previous systems. To achieve the highest possible sensitivities, the electronics can be cooled with liquid nitrogen. Ultra-high resolution (2,048 × 2,048 pixels) CCDs are now commercially available and even higher resolution chips with 4,096 × 4,096 pixels are being developed.

A schematic drawing of the measurement possibilities by optical methods is illustrated in Figure 10.5. A rectangular array of equally spaced pixels is a convenient format for digital analysis. Either the light intensity or the rate of light intensity change with time (quenching lifetime) can be quantified for each pixel. The image can be displayed as a gray level scale as illustrated in Figure 10.5, or pseudo-colored images can be generated which are often easier to interpret by visual inspection. Using the newest generation of CCDs, it will be possible to have resolutions of 12 bits per pixel (4,096 gray levels). The individual scan lines for a captured image can be analyzed and a frequency distribution of analyte concentrations at a specific location or across a region of the image can be obtained, as illustrated for two scan lines in Figure 10.5. The heterogeneous distribution of concentrations for the entire image can also be compiled. Temporal changes can be determined by comparing sequential scans for a particular location or for the whole image.

Multiple dye interference coatings are being developed to improve the bandpass filtering of optical components. Efficiencies on the order of 75% are possible at the present time. Further advances can be expected, and many more optical applications will be developed taking advantage of the wide dynamic ranges and broad spectral sensitivity of CCDs. Detailed spatial and temporal information could be derived from optical fibers coupled to CCDs for use with optical biosensors.

10.5.2 CCD Spectrophotometry

Cope et al. (1989) described an application of a liquid nitrogen–cooled CCD array detector with 385 horizontal and 578 vertical elements for noninvasive measurements in the near-infrared range in living tissues. They studied the brains of anesthetized rats, and obtained spectra for oxyhemoglobin and deoxygenated hemoglobin, for cytochrome a,a_3, and for water. Some animals were completely blood transfusion–exchanged with a perfluorocarbon blood substitute to reduce the possible interference of hemoglobin with the cytochrome a,a_3 signal. Similar optical technology using CCD detectors will be developed for human noninvasive monitoring under clinical situations.

10.5.3 Noninvasive Phosphorescence Measurements

Wilson et al. (1987) have utilized the quenching by O_2 on the phosphorescence lifetime of the lumiphore palladium coproporphyrin to study O_2 metabolism in isolated mitochondria. The technique was quickly applied to *in vivo* measurements in animals and *in vitro* measurements in perfused organs, as described by Rumsey et al. (1988). Palladium coproporphyrin binds to blood plasma proteins and can remain in the bloodstream for long times. The phosphorescence was measured after a flash from a xenon arc lamp. This technology could be easily adapted to fiberoptic or waveguide measurements with lumiphores as the phosphorescent source at the tip. Clinically, the intravascular PO_2 could be measured noninvasively during various surgical procedures, or examined on a diagnostic basis in the choroidal and retinal circulation of the eye, or in the skin. Nontoxic phosphorescent dyes and their carrier systems will need the U.S. Food and Drug Administration's (FDA) approval before this technology is adopted for human use.

10.5.4 Artificial Eyes

Miyasaka et al. (1992), a team of Japanese scientists at the Fuji Film Company, recently developed an ultra-thin film with bacteriorhodopsin fragments which they coated over an SnO_2 conductive surface to create a photocell. Robert Birge at the University of Syracuse has also fabricated light-sensitive devices with the same bacterial protein pigment. The SnO_2 layer, deposited 4,500 Å thick on a glass plate, was optically transparent. The film was applied by the Langmuir-Blodgett method, and was 50 to 500 Å thick, depending on the number of layers. An aqueous gel electrolyte containing 1 M KCl was then coated over the film with a 200 μm thick Teflon ring spacer. The SnO_2 electrode, gel, and spacer were then sand-wiched next to an Au-coated glass plate. A negative bias voltage between 0 to -0.7 was applied between the Au electrode and the electrically grounded SnO_2 electrode. Transient photocurrents were generated with response times < 300 μsecond when light was switched on or off. This meant that the photocell responded to changes in light intensity rather than to light intensity alone. The logarithm of the change in photocurrent density, which ranged from about 1 nanoampere to 1 μampere per cm^2, was linear with the logarithm of the change in light intensity ranging from about 10^{-4} to 10^{-1} W/cm^2. This property of the photocell means that it operates as a differential transducer, ignoring the constant background or ambient light and allowing easier detection of moving images. Tests on the quantum efficiency of the film were conducted using electrochemical techniques. The efficiency was found to be on the order of 0.01. Although this value is small, the device was much more efficient than other devices that have attempted to use bacteriorhodopsin.

A small (2.5 mm by 2.5 mm) "artificial eye" was constructed from a 64 pixel array of photolithographed indium-tin oxide electrodes coated with the bacteriorhodopsin film, electrolyte gel, and common electrode (Au). The "eye" was tested using a slide projector to project images of simple letters onto the array. Since the photocell does not respond to steady light intensities, the images were modulated between 20 to 50 Hz using a simple mechanical light chopper. The signals from each indium-tin oxide electrode were amplified and used to drive LEDs to duplicate the received image. This relatively simple device was capable of many functions that are accomplished by more complicated electronic devices, and could be a low-cost visual sensor for industrial robots. Many other image processing applications may be possible with this type of photocell, with perhaps some applications for biosensors.

10.5.5 Chemically Tuned LEDs

Burn et al. (1992) recently described enhanced quantum yields for poly(p-phenylenevinylene) electroluminescent copolymers. The ratio of conjugated and nonconjugated polymers could be controlled, so the color of the emission in the yellow-green wavelengths could be varied. The polymerization methods appear to be readily adaptable to photolithographic processes, and might permit precise tuning of the emitted wavelength, or creation of patterns with different emission wavelengths.

10.5.6 Enzymes under Glass

Ellerby et al. (1992) recently reported a technique for making new types of transparent porous silicate glasses that are able to encapsulate enzymes while retaining their native spectroscopic properties and their normal bioactivity. As has been previously described, it is difficult to maintain the stability and long-term bioactivity of enzymes in many types of biosensors. Normal methods of immobilizing the enzymes may greatly contribute to the degradation in their performance. A silica glass was prepared by a sol-gel method, where the alkoxide $Si(OCH_3)_4$ (tetramethylorthosilicate) was mixed with HCl in a methanol solvent. After forming the glass, a buffer was added to bring the pH above five, then enzymes were encapsulated into the aggregate mixture. Excess methanol was avoided to minimize its effects on denaturing the enzymes. Three enzymes — copper-zinc superoxide dismutase, horse heart cytochrome c, and horse heart myoglobin — were tested. All of these enzymes have well-known spectral properties and very high O_2 affinities, so they are very sensitive at low O_2. After mixing, the mixture was hardened by allowing the solvent to evaporate. The dry gel volume typically dropped to about 1/8 of the original volume, further concentrating the enzyme. The resulting dried gel is rigid and optically transparent, with fine pore networks (< 100 Å) that allow diffusion of small molecules without appreciable light scattering. The optical spectra measured for these three glass-encapsulated enzymes were similar to spectra measured for the enzymes in aqueous solutions. The authors also mentioned that they had tested some other enzymes, including glucose oxidase, peroxidase, chymotrypsin, and trypsin, and also found that they all remained enzymatically active after encapsulation in glass. It is very probable that optical biosensors will be developed in the near future using this new type of glass-encapsulated enzyme.

10.6 ADVANCES IN ENZYME AND PROTEIN ENGINEERING

Although there are critics of the current trends in genetic manipulation of living organisms by recombinant DNA techniques, and concerns about efforts to directly manipulate human genes, it is clear that the technological advances in this area will continue to accelerate. The National Institutes of Health has filed two patent applications so far for literally thousands of human gene fragments and is expected to submit another application soon for thousands more. NIH researcher Craig Venter, using automated gene sequencing instruments, has been averaging 168 gene fragment isolations per day. There has been concern and debate about the ethics of these patent claims, since the characteristics and functions of each gene fragment are not fully known. The task of completely characterizing all of the human genes could take decades. Future licensing by industry for specific gene applications could become problematic, as well as international in scope. There are fears that there will be an era of secrecy or restricted scientific exchange, delaying the potential therapeutic applications that are anticipated from the Human Genome Project.

Whatever the outcome of this huge scientific effort, it is clear that we are living in a era of designer genes and synthetic proteins. For example, Schnölzer and Kent (1992) recently reported the synthesis of a totally engineered HIV protease. The protease was completely chemically synthesized in high yields, and was found to be fully active. The chemical synthesis techniques are readily adapted to other proteins, and hybrids of proteins with other molecules. Customized enzymes and other biologically active molecules are likely to be developed in the near future, which will have many practical applications. New techniques for producing monoclonal and polyclonal antibodies will also be developed and utilized for immunosensors. Sustained release polymer-based drug delivery systems are also of great practical importance. A new hyperbranched dendrimer polymer is receiving attention as a possible drug delivery system. Tomalia (1990) discovered a way to control the size and number of units in these polymers. Hollow, spherical polymers with diameters between 95 and 105 Å may be useful for crossing cell membranes, if they can internalize and release therapeutically useful drugs. They would be much smaller than current liposome carriers. As illustrated by some of the examples discussed in this book, some of these new technologies have already become integrated into biosensor designs.

10.7 PROJECTIONS FOR FOOD AND BEVERAGE INDUSTRIES

The food processing industry is an area where it is anticipated that there will be increasing commercial applications for biosensors to monitor the quality of different production methods. Microbial toxins, such as mycotoxins that can contaminate milk, peanuts, corn, and wheat, can already be detected by enzyme-linked immunosorbent assays or by radioimmunoassay methods. It may prove to be more cost-effective to use biosensors for these tests. Another area where biosensors are expected to be useful is in the monitoring of bioprocessing reactors for synthetic foods. Synthetic foods and food additive industries have already grown to a $5.5 billion market in the United States (Thayer, 1991).

10.8 PROJECTIONS FOR DEFENSE SECTOR

Biosensors for detecting chemical warfare agents, nerve gases, and other toxic agents are of interest to the defense industry. The piezoelectric microbalance or surface acoustic wave transducers have been investigated for possible use as air sampling chemical noses. A neural network type of pattern recognition approach might be incorporated into the design to provide early warning biosensor systems built into aircraft and mobile vehicles to detect noxious gases in the external air. Of course, the level of research funding for the military may be deeply cut and biosensor-oriented research may be limited.

10.9 PROJECTIONS FOR ENVIRONMENTAL APPLICATIONS

Biosensors are beginning to have applications for the analysis of environmental contaminants, where simple, reliable assays of air, water, or soil samples that can be conducted quickly in the field are needed. Immunosensors may be the most useful biosensors for this purpose. Van Emon and Lopez-Avila (1992) have reviewed some of the field portable immunoassays used by the U.S. Environmental Protection Agency that can effectively identify environmental contaminants. Specific antibodies have already been developed for a number of pesticides and industrial wastes. Most of the current monitoring instruments use either enzyme-linked immunosorbent assays or radioimmunoassay methods. The latter technique is not portable and is the most expensive laboratory method. Future developments in biosensors may allow more cost-effective and portable monitoring of contaminated sites and expedite their cleanup by monitoring the progress of bioremediation procedures.

10.10 PROJECTIONS FOR MEDICAL INSTRUMENTS INDUSTRY

There are several clinical areas that might benefit from the availability of many different types of biosensors that so far have been limited to experimental research. The medical monitoring and diagnostic instrument industries are expected to be the largest potential users of new biosensors. In 1991, the U.S. medical instruments industries exported approximately $3.8 billion more in medical instruments than the U.S. imported. Advances in biosensors will have a positive impact on exports.

A variety of types of bedside monitors could be specifically programmed using replaceable biosensors for detecting analytes in the blood, cerebral spinal fluid, urine, or other medical samples. Heart attack and stroke victims might be more reliably treated during the most acute stages of their recovery by monitoring creatinine, lactic acid, and other biochemical analytes in the blood. Genetic and diagnostic testing could be facilitated by biosensors. Noninvasive optical technologies, as discussed earlier in this chapter, are expected to be available in the near future.

10.11 PROJECTIONS FOR BIOTECHNOLOGY AND PHARMACEUTICAL INDUSTRIES

The biotechnology industry was initially a phenomenon in the United States, with an initially rapid rate of growth that produced literally hundreds of companies in the early 1980s. Many of these companies were very successful in transferring new biotechnology techniques (e.g., monoclonal antibodies, recombinant DNA) to create new drugs. Since 1975, the U.S. pharmaceuticals industry has been responsible for developing 47 of the 97 major new drugs that have been introduced into world markets.

However, there are enormous expenses and lengthy procedures for testing and receiving FDA approval for new pharmaceutical products, which can take 10 to 12 years before they reach the marketplace. This has taken its toll. A recent report from the Office of Technology Assessment (*Biotechnology in a Global Economy*, OTA-BA-494, October, 1991) names only 46 biotechnology companies that are still currently listed on the security exchanges. Clinical applications of biotechnology began with the production of insulin by implanting human genes in bacteria. Bioreactor-produced insulin reached the market in 1982. Recombinant DNA technology saw its first entry in the marketplace with the introduction of human growth hormone, reaching $250 million in sales in 1988. Currently, there are around 100 biotechnology-based drugs that have been submitted for the FDA approval process. Most of these drugs are designed for treating cancer, and some could be of benefit in treating AIDS. As of May, 1991 the FDA had approved only 15 biotechnology-based drugs. Although there have been great expectations for the development of new drugs, out of the estimated $150 billion in worldwide pharmaceutical sales at the present time, less than $1 billion directly involves the biotechnology industries. That low percentage is very likely to increase in the next few years. The pharmaceuticals industry is presently devoting about 16% of current sales revenue into new research.

The licensing of biotechnology products in Europe as it moves toward the single market concept has been significantly streamlined. The licensing procedure is often more efficient and quicker than that used by the U.S. FDA. Of the 135 new drugs approved by the FDA between 1984 and 1989, a total of 106 were first approved in other countries. The past year (1991) has been described as a banner economic year for European biotechnology firms. In the U.S., a presidential Biotechnology Research Initiative was announced as part of the 1993 federal budget. This appears to be an attempt to coordinate biotechnology-related expenditures through 12 federal agencies. According to information released at a press conference in January, 1992 by Allen Bromley, director of the White House Office of Science and Technology Policy, biotechnology funding will increase by 7% to a total of $4.03 billion. Over half ($2.94 billion) will be administered through the National Institutes of Health. However, there have been concerns expressed that the U.S. does not have a national policy, and regulatory issues are not being addressed.

A recent market projection by Consulting Resources Corp. (Lexington, MA) for biosensors used in the bioprocessing industry alone estimates sales of $50 million by 1995 and $250 million by the year 2000 (*Chemical Engineering Progress*, January, 1992).

10.12 REFERENCES

Aoki, A., T. Matsue and I. Uchida. 1992. "Multichannel Electrochemical Detection with a Microelectrode Array in Flowing Streams," *Anal. Chem.*, 64:44–49.

Bard, A. J., F-R. F. Fan, D. T. Pierce, P. R. Unwin, D. O. Wipf and F. Zhou. 1991. "Chemical Imaging of Surfaces with the Scanning Electrochemical Microscope," *Science Wash. DC*, 254:68–80.

Buerk, D. G. and T. K. Goldstick. 1982. "Arterial Wall Oxygen Consumption Rate Varies Spatially," *Am. J. Physiol.*, 243:H948–H958.

Buerk, D. G. and T. K. Goldstick. In press. "Spatial Variation of Aortic Wall Oxygen Diffusion Coefficient from Transient Polarographic Measurements," *Annals Biomed. Eng.*

Buerk, D. G. and G. M. Saidel. 1978. "Local Kinetics of Oxygen Metabolism in Brain and Liver Tissues," *Microvas. Res.*, 16:391–405.

Buerk, D. G., L. Hoofd and Z. Turek. 1989. "Microelectrode Studies of Facilitated O_2 Transport across Hemoglobin and Myoglobin Layers," in *Oxygen Transport to Tissue—XI*, K.

Rakusan, G. P. Biro, T. K. Goldstick and Z. Turek, eds., New York, NY: Plenum Press; *Adv. Exp. Med. & Biol.*, 248:125–135.

Buerk, D. G., C. E. Riva, R. D. Shonat and S. D. Cranstoun. 1992. "Optic Nerve Head Blood Flow, PO_2 and K^+ Dynamics during Diffuse Luminance Flicker Stimulus," *Invest. Ophthalmol. Vis. Sci.*, 33(abstract):1939.

Buerk, D. G., R. D. Shonat and C. E. Riva. In press. "O_2 Gradients and Countercurrent Exchange in the Cat Vitreous Humor near Retinal Arterioles and Veins," *Microvas. Res.*

Burn, P. L., A. B. Holmes, A. Kraft, D. D. C. Bradley, A. R. Brown, R. H. Friend and R. W. Gymer. 1992. "Chemical Tuning of Electroluminescent Copolymers to Improve Emission Efficiencies and Allow Patterning," *Nature*, 356:47–49.

Cope, M., D. T. Delpy, S. Wray, J. S. Wyatt and E. O. R. Reynolds. 1989. "A CCD Spectrophotometer to Quantitate the Concentration of Chromophores in Living Tissue Utilising the Absorption Peak of Water at 975 nm," in *Oxygen Transport to Tissue—IX*, K. Rakusan, G. P. Biro, T. K. Goldstick and Z. Turek, eds., New York, NY: Plenum Press; *Adv. Exp. Med. & Biol.*, 248:33–40.

Ellerby, L. M., C. R. Nishida, F. Nishida, S. A. Yamanaka, B. Dunn, J. Selverstone-Valentine and J. I. Zink. 1992. "Encapsulation of Proteins in Transparent Porous Silicate Glasses Prepared by the Sol-Gel Method," *Science Wash. D.C.*, 255:1113–1115.

Miyasaka, T., K. Koyama and I. Itoh. 1992. "Quantum Conversion and Image Detection by a Bacteriorhodopsin-Based Artificial Photoreceptor," *Science Wash. DC*, 255:342–344.

Pournaras, C. J., R. D. Shonat, J-L. Munoz and B. L. Petrig. 1991. "New Ocular Micromanipulator for Measurements of Retinal and Vitreous Physiologic Parameters in the Mammalian Eye," *Exp. Eye Res.*, 53:23–27.

Roh, H-D., T. K. Goldstick and R. A. Linsenmeier. 1990. "Spatial Variation of the Local Tissue Oxygen Diffusion Coefficient Measured In Situ in the Cat Retina and Cornea," in *Oxygen Transport to Tissue—XII*. J. Piiper, T. K. Goldstick and M. Meyer, eds., New York, NY: Plenum Press; *Adv. Exp. Med. & Biol.*, 277:127–136.

Rumsey, W. L., J. M. Vanderkooi and D. F. Wilson. 1988. "Imaging of Phosphorescence: A Novel Method for Measuring Oxygen Distribution in Perfused Tissue," *Science Wash. DC*, 241:1649–1651.

Schnölzer, M. and S. B. H. Kent. 1992. "Constructing Proteins by Dovetailing Unprotected Synthetic Peptides: Backbone-Engineering HIV Protease," *Science Wash. DC*, 256:221–225.

Thayer, A. M. 1991. "Use of Specialty Food Additives Continues to Grow," *Chem. Eng. News*, 69:9–12.

Tomalia, D. A., A. M. Naylor and W. A. Goddard, III. 1990. "Starburst Dendimers: Molecular-Level Control of Size, Shape, Surface Chemistry, Topology, and Flexibility from Atoms to Macroscopic Matter," *Angew. Chemie*, 29:138–175.

Van Emon, J. M. and V. Lopez-Avila. 1992. "Immunochemical Methods for Environmental Analysis," *Anal. Chem.*, 64:79A–88A.

Wilson, D. F., W. L. Rumsey, T. J. Green and J. M. Vanderkooi. 1988. "The Oxygen Dependence of Mitochondrial Oxidative Phosphorylation Measured by a New Optical Method for Measuring Oxygen Concentration," *J. Biol. Chem.*, 263:2712–2718.

217

Donald G. Buerk was born in St. Louis, Missouri in 1946. His professional training is in biomedical and chemical engineering. He received a B.S. degree in engineering from Case Western Reserve University, Cleveland, Ohio in 1969. After graduation, he was a biomedical engineer in Dr. William J. Whalen's research laboratory at St. Vincent Charity Hospital in Cleveland, Ohio for six years. He received an M.S. degree in biomedical engineering from Case Western Reserve University in 1976, and a Ph.D. in chemical engineering from Northwestern University, Evanston, Illinois in 1980. He began his academic career in the Department of Biomedical Engineering at Louisiana Technical University, Ruston, Louisiana in 1982. In 1986, he was a Visiting Professor in the laboratory of Richard J. Traystman in the Department of Anesthesiology at The Johns Hopkins University School of Medicine, Baltimore, Maryland, where he still holds an honorary appointment. In 1987, he joined the Biomedical Engineering and Science Institute at Drexel University in Philadelphia, Pennsylvania. In 1988, he was a Visiting Scientist at Catholic University in Nijmegen, the Netherlands. He joined the Department of Ophthalmology and the Institute for Environmental Medicine at the University of Pennsylvania School of Medicine, Philadelphia, Pennsylvania in 1990. Dr. Buerk's primary research interests include mathematical modeling of biotransport phenomena, oxygen transport and metabolism, and the regulation of blood flow. He is presently developing new electrochemical microbiosensors for physiological measurements in the eye, brain, carotid body, and other tissues. His research is funded by grants from the National Science Foundation and the National Institutes of Health.